A Companion to Medical Statistics

The Johns Hopkins Series in Contemporary Medicine and Public Health

A Companion to Medical Statistics

Edmond A. Murphy, M.D.

THE JOHNS HOPKINS UNIVERSITY PRESS
Baltimore and London

The Johns Hopkins University Press, 701 West 40th Street, Baltimore, Maryland 21211
The Johns Hopkins Press Ltd, London

The paper in this book is acid-free and meets the guidelines for permanence and durability of the Committee on Production Guidelines for Book Longevity of the Council on Library Resources.

Illustrations by the author

Library of Congress Cataloging in Publication Data

Murphy, Edmond A., 1925–
    A companion to medical statistics.

    Bibliography: p.
    Includes index.
    1. Medical statistics.   2. Biometry.   I. Title. [DNLM: 1. Biometry. 2. Statistics.
WA 950 M978c] RA409.M868 1985   574′.072   84-21806
ISBN 0-8018-2612-8 (alk. paper)

*For Madi M. and Madi R., Manolo, Cathi,
Micky, Marcos, Mary, and Edmond—
a set of sufficient genotypes*

Contents

Preface

There seems to be a clear difference between the needs of those who do research and write and those who read medical literature as a source of knowledge. The consumer (if I may be pardoned the vulgarity of the term) needs to know how to tell sound scholarship from bad; what the results mean; and how they may be responsibly applied. The supplier, as it were, is obliged to know not merely much more detail, but detail of a different kind. Medical students suffer much because we have failed to distinguish between these two demands. We still design the medical curriculum as if, after four brief years, the graduate should not only have professional competence in all the basic sciences but also be clinically equipped to undertake anything from a psychoanalysis to an amputation of a hindquarter. Now while nobody, in fact, believes this myth, a kind of vestigial homage is paid to it by imparting not merely broad knowledge (which has merit) but also detail, detail that is often insufficient for professional purposes, but quite sufficient to confuse the student. I cannot imagine what is to be gained from learning to do something complicated—a karyotype or an electropheresis—not only without skill but without dedicated interest or comprehension.

Statisticians are among the biggest sinners in their lack of perspective. I have sat through many statistics lectures to medical students on such topics as the incomplete gamma integral, confidence limits on sample estimates of the variance, the Behrens-Fisher problem, and the chi-square approximation to the F variate. When young and foolish (May I be forgiven!), I even participated in teaching such courses to them myself. Within the last year I have seen a question set in an examination for medical students that could be solved only by a two-way analysis of variance after stabilizing the variance by a suitable transformation. I have seen too many students sulkily cramming their heads with such detail, reproducing it in garbled form at examinations, and being left later in life with nothing whatsoever but painful scars from the experience. Such a lamentable outcome is only to be expected in most of them (even if a few mathematically gifted students come through the statistical ordeal unscathed and even with some enrichment).

Nonetheless there is no dispute that a physician must know a good deal about assessing evidence. Doing so with what the patient tells him is a large part of his clinical training. How to evaluate the performance of a new diagnostic test—an issue that arises more and more frequently—receives much less attention. Students are encouraged to read the current literature, but not always to read it critically, and too often they have been given no equipment for doing so. They rarely have it pointed out to them that world experts in high-resolution basic sciences who turn their hands to medical applications may make crass errors, through ignorance of sampling methods or through failure to distinguish random variation from a systematic effect. All inference calls for ideas and methods. But in order to cultivate discernment rather than virtuosity, clear ideas are incomparably more important than technique. Often, all that is needed is the skill to ask the right question in plain prose. To see the unconscious humor in a statement will often take the sting out of a lesson. I have recently heard a statement on the radio: "Cases of armed robbery increased 20 percent last year. The police attribute this increase to the recent crime wave." There is nothing, one feels, like discerning analysis by the expert mind.

Many of the scarred warriors of student classes cannot altogether forget. Some retain an illusory sense of loss. I call it illusory because though they know there is something missing, it is not a loss of anything they have ever been given. I hazard the guess that nobody has explained to them what may, and may not, be inferred from a bimodal distribution; or the pros and cons of classification and its alternatives; or the evidential importance of meaning. These are issues that lie at the heart of everyday medicine. They are not (in my opinion) the philosophy of medicine, which is best left to the experts in that field. In the ideal world they would be part of that already overburdened subject, pathology. Indeed, facets of it are touched on in the better books on clinical pathology. They mostly fall outside the canon of statistics, largely because statistics, even biostatistics, is becoming progressively more formalized.

While I would aim to heighten the critical perception of the reader, I know from experience that there are two big dangers in doing so. The first is that a kind of supercilious skepticism may result. The aims of being critical are, not to deride and to demolish, but to develop an authentic habit of appreciation. The content and form of a paper may leave much to be desired; nevertheless, it may contain by far the best information to date on some particular topic. We should not swallow it whole; yet we may be far wiser after reading it than beforehand. Rough truth is better than precise ignorance. Nevertheless, the critical mind, however appreciative, will never lose sight of the fact that it is only rough truth.

The other danger is superficiality. The thought of the age is beset by two dangerous patterns: that it is better to read extensively than intensively and that all precision is numerical or factual. The first explains the popularity of courses in rapid reading rather than in condensed writing. The second explains the neglect of critical reading and the popularity of what purport to be courses on science. The student is tempted to leaf through a book dealing with ideas, nod at a few randomly chosen sentences, and fancy that he is ready to do a stiff examination on its contents and their applications. Studying any book word by word is out of fashion. Should he have to read a sentence three times to understand it fully, he is apt to complain about the obscurity of the style. If he has to look up the meaning of a word (perhaps a word chosen with excruciating care to avoid ambiguity or longwinded paraphrase), he will dismiss the writing as pedantic or tortured. Common sense is his greatest asset in critical reading; but common sense—like a sense of rhythm, or literary style—must be cultivated. They are rarely effortless native talents.

In this book I propose to cater to some of the needs of the clinical spectator. I imply no slight by this term. I am not patronizing readers. If they had an indefinite amount of time available, I am sure they could master formal analysis in any amount of detail. I am thinking rather of people who are interested in knowledge because they perceive it as important, but who have no ambitions to set up as investigating scientists or as professional critics. I have devoted more than my share of effort to meeting the needs of the latter group.

Who are included among these "clinicians?" Anybody at all who has to do with the living patient: physicians, surgeons, dentists, veterinarians, nurses, medical students, psychologists, human geneticists, social workers, even enterprising lawyers, pharmacists, and clergy. Anybody, in a word, who has need of some insight into the issues of science as applied to the care of the living. I have tried to keep the many examples simple, with brief explanatory notes as need be. I do not want an illustration bypassed because it calls for too much background. I have avoided calculations wherever possible.

ABOUT THIS BOOK

I have arranged the three sections of this book in the order in which the subject matter occurs to most students. Before we get to the middle section, which deals with the formal ideas and methods of inference, we must give some thought to what it is we try to do by those methods. The first section is called "Perspective"; this ominous term need cause no alarm. It is an attempt to see how far words and ideas, rather than algebra and calculation, help us to understand evidence and how to interpret it. Even in the second section, "Probability and Statistics," I am much more concerned with the strategies (that is, broad, long-term plans in perspective) than the tactics (the equipment for dealing with immediate problems). Elementary treatments of these topics commonly become so bogged down in technical detail and calculations that, even after much studying and acquiring some formal agility, the reader may have gained little insight into what the broad objectives are. Some few notes on formal technique are relegated to the appropriate place, an appendix. Like most patients, the main intent of this book will readily survive an appendectomy.

The second section leaves unfinished business. For in exploring the principles of evidence, venturesome clinicians may curb their impatience for the time being and sally forth from the comfortable world of concrete detail into the rather bleak world of theory. They do so on the promise of better and deeper understanding. But at the end of it all, they wish to translate the conclusions back into terms of the concrete reality with which they are familiar. I think it is a capital error to underrate the importance or the difficulties of this last step of translating back. It is getting increasingly difficult to practice good medicine without a knowledge of biochemistry. But for the clinician, the subject of biochemistry is an artificial abstraction. Conclusions from test-tube studies cannot at once and without thoughtful modification be applied to a patient in a bed. The discerning physician will adapt his knowledge, knowing where it will serve and where it will mislead. A clinical problem converted into a biochemical mode to find a solution must, when solved, be *faithfully* translated back into clinical terms. I am saying exactly the same about both probability and statistics. So I have a third section that addresses this problem. I have few fears that physicians will be seduced by incongruous arguments where the clinical details are secure: in tuberculosis or gout or an avitaminosis. But the dangers are immense in a clinically confused field, when the clinician is casting around for guidance from another discipline and guilelessly supposes that immunology, or genetics, epidemiology or statistics, has authoritative, ready-made, answers. It is in these vulnerable areas of translation that I wish to provide safeguards.

I furnish a brief glossary of terms, which I trust will be consulted and used with the precision that I have aimed to give it.

Finally, the problems. I have not (as I have done in my other books) furnished model answers. Those who think about the problems a little will discover more often than not that what they should be focusing on is not the answer (which is usually easy to find and often trivial) but the question. Like the outcome of a conjuring trick, the obvious answer may not be the truth but the result of subtle misdirection in the question. Some of the problems (e.g., 1.1, 6.3, 11.1) are facetious. What is to be learnt from them is, not whether the obvious answer is right, but how the readers have been trapped into giving a fatuous answer and how they may easily be misled when the fatuity is less blatant.

Acknowledgments

I am grateful to my colleagues Drs. Paul Whelton, Dennis Noe, and Jorge Sequeiros, E. C. Foster and three anonymous reviewers, who have read this text in detail; and to Drs. C. L. Conley, D. F. Proctor, G. W. Thorn, and K. D. Smith, who have clarified individual points. They have all helped to keep me from errors of fact, taste, and judgment. No blame attaches to them for remaining flaws. Dr. P. O. Kwiterovich kindly furnished the data for figure 10.3. The editors of *The Johns Hopkins Medical Journal* and *The American Journal of Medical Genetics* have graciously allowed me to reproduce figures 3.3 and 7.3, respectively.

Part **❚** | Perspective

1 | Sound Generalization: Subject and Scope

Any organized field needs sound generalizations. This first chapter will say something about how they are to be attained, and their limits to be defined. The most widely read part of any paper is the title, which is an important factor in determining which readers will be attracted to it. But publicity apart, the title is important because *it defines the scope* of the paper. However, the title is not an abstract. If long, it is apt to repel.

The author must play fair. The title is as much a scientific statement as the text itself; and while an inaccurate title may be corrected by more circumspect statements in the text, it is still apt to mislead and, if so, perhaps to leave the unfortunate impression of deliberate dishonesty. The sound scholar makes good the promises given or implied in the title. If the title of the paper is "Survivorship in Primary Atypical Pneumonia," it will not do to find half a page later that the analysis is based on a series of necropsies; for (one hopes) the subjects then consist exclusively of patients who have not survived. I can recall a paper with a title (that I shall diplomatically disguise as) "A New Index for Predicting Myocardial Infarction," in which the cases were middle-aged men recovering from heart attacks and the controls were children. I can think of much easier ways of distinguishing middle-aged men from children than by complicated analysis of blood lipid fractions. In any case, it is hardly appropriate to proclaim the *predictive* value of the index when the subjects had already developed myocardial infarction. For what is then observed may be the result of the disorder and not a precursor of it.

Usually, I am sure, this kind of distortion is not intentionally misleading but is instead symptomatic of a general vagueness in the minds of the writers as to what problem they are addressing. If the reader is to gain anything from a paper, there are several issues that must be explicitly decided before the work is even undertaken.

THE POPULATION OF REFERENCE

To what group are the results of the study being ascribed? It will be obvious that the effects of sex hormones are apt to be different in men and in women; that growth hormone will have different impacts before and after the growing parts of the bone are sealed off; that certain genetic diseases are commoner in some racial groups than in others; that certain occupations carry peculiar risks. The critical reader will look for clear statements about the scope of the study, and the sound investigator will furnish them. Nowadays, there seems little to be said for vague generalizations about haphazard collections of reminiscences, however exquisitely observed. Studies dealing with opportunistic research (such as those on rare diseases) are necessarily of this kind. The medical geneticist cannot order forty patients with (say) mucolipidosis type IV as the laboratory geneticist can make such an order for C57Black mice. The scientist must depend on happy accidents and use ingenuity and penetration of analysis to redress their haphazard origins. Description has its problems. But experimentation is another matter. Too often, vague papers are due to vague experiments that are not prompted by any coherent approach to an explicit problem. A common instance is the newly devised test or machine, for which the enthusiast can see a thousand possible uses and rashly tries to fulfill all of them simultaneously in a handful of patients.

The reaction to my criticisms may be that they are harsh for so small a fault. Harsh, yes. But how serious the fault is depends on how much the reader is misled. However, it is useless to talk about how misleading a conclusion may be unless it is clear, at least in principle, what the true answer would be if the right information were to hand. And here the trouble begins. Let us try to address the problem systematically.

The first requirement is an explicit statement about what the *universe* or *population* or *reference set* may be. It is surprising how many people do not raise this question until after the data have been collected. Indeed, it is surprising how many people never raise it or state it at all. If I were to ask "Should candidates for admission to medical school be selected on the basis of color?" I daresay there would be an immediate outcry. Color has nothing to do with performance. But that is nonsense. If, in self-justification, I point out that a candidate with red petals and yellow stamens should not be admitted, the protestors will be forced to agree; but they will complain that I have tricked them. However, it is their business to find out what my population of reference was if I have not had the good grace to state it expressly. I never said that the choice was limited to human beings: That was a reasonable, but gratuitous, assumption on the part of the listener. I can balance my statement that I have never personally known an intelligent Eskimo, with the wider claim that I have never personally known an Eskimo at all. The proportion of people in a particular racial group admitted to college is no test of bigotry; for incidental differences may mean that (because of a higher birth rate, for instance) the underrepresented group contain disproportionately many people too young to go to college. However, the implication would be quite different if the reference set were properly defined as those of college age that have the necessary academic qualifications.

SAMPLING AND RANDOM SAMPLING

The most obvious way of making a sound general statement about some trait in a defined population is to obtain the information on every member and to tabulate the results. This method is used in certain cases: in a census, in an election, or in the study of rare, but conspicuous, disorders. There are two main groups of reasons why one abandons this method in favor of a method of sampling that is no longer exhaustive.

The first is the obvious one that an exhaustive search may be a prohibitive task: too expensive; too slow for prompt action; in some cases to take the entire population (such as all of a patient's blood!) would be ethically indefensible.

The second reason is more subtle. Diagnosis of a patient's disease is a clinical and personal activity; it becomes related to science only because there is a real, or supposed, rational connection between a disease and its signs, which is established by evidence acquired from all such patients and applicable to each. At the heart of scientific enquiry lies *generalization*. The knowledge that twenty-seven patients called (let us say) Marshbanks in West Virginia suffer from Dinglewhizzit's syndrome is in itself little more than gossip. It may lead to the discovery that this disease is genetic; but in itself it is of no scientific interest, because family names (being arbitrary) do not come within the ambit of science. If all such patients had the same blood group, the fact might be used as an interesting illustration of (say) genetic drift. But unless it meant something wider, the scientist would not be interested. This series of twenty-seven cases, particularly if they include all cases in the reference population, can mean nothing to other clinicians unless it has some bearing on patients they themselves have some chance of seeing.

• *Always, scientific fact has the implication that it is relevant to a larger and wider group than that on which it was established.*

These two basic notions (sampling and generalizability) bear on how to interpret one's samples, even when they are taken from the same reference set. I may wish to treat my own reference set as the object of enquiry—let us say that I am interested in patients from Baltimore only. Then its finiteness must always be kept in mind. A modest size in the reference set will call for adjustment in the estimates.

Example 1.1. To find the prevalence of tuberculosis in Baltimore, I must realize that as each person is examined and "crossed off the list," the composition of the population still eligible for sampling changes, and this systematic change must be taken into account in analysis.

But if I see my task as finding the prevalence of tuberculosis in a population (arguably an infinite population) of which Baltimore is seen as merely an intermediate sample,* I may ignore this refinement. The reader may feel—and with warrant—that this way of viewing the data is rather contrived. But it is much more akin to the nature of scientific statements. Nobody objects to the physicist discussing what would happen if two stars with particular specifications were to approach one another on particular courses that brought them close to each other. The actual event may have been observed only a few times; it may have happened any number of times. But while the physicist welcomes empirical† experience, nobody would suggest that the relationship between the laws of physics and the behavior of the stars depends on the sample size. While the argument must not be abused, I still hold that the scientific interest (as distinct, say, from the political and public-health interest) in the prevalence of tuberculosis in Baltimore is vitiated if we cannot see it as one outcome of an event that might, in principle, occur any number of times.

---

*This notion raises certain subtleties that will be addressed later.

†To avoid misunderstandings, the reader may wish to consult the exact meanings given in the glossary for words that are unfamiliar or that seem to be used in an unusual sense.

The preferred method of selection is known technically as *random sampling*. We shall describe it shortly. The idea is to select a set of members of a population in such a way that sound probabilistic inferences can be made from it. The word *random* is an unfortunate one because, in common usage, the only images it produces are vagueness, capriciousness, a total lack of system. The lay mind does not distinguish it from *chaotic* or *haphazard*. To avoid this confusion, some scientific writers talk about "probability sampling," a nicer term, but one that, unfortunately, has never become popular. In any case, the technical use of the terms *random* and *randomness* is so fundamental that the discerning reader must eventually come to grips with it.

The term *random* is so commonly misused that the *reader is expressly warned not to take at face value unqualified statements in a scientific study that the sample studied was random.* If the writer does not state explicitly the method of randomization or random sampling used we should fear the worst. There are many more-or-less elaborate schemes of random sampling according to what properties are required of the sample. These, too, should be specified. The topic is large and technical, and I can aim for no more than a brief outline here.

One could write a long cautionary essay on how *not* to collect a random sample. It does *not* mean any of the following: (1) that the writer has no clear idea how the subjects came to be chosen; (2) that no plan was followed in picking them; (3) that no class is *known* to have been discriminated for or against; (4) that it is difficult to see why the cases should not be representative. The issue of randomness must be addressed and planned beforehand, and must not be assumed on the basis of a historical reconstruction afterwards of how the scientist thinks he may have found his cases.

Now to business. Let us begin with a definition.

DEFINITION. *A random (probability) sample is one chosen from a* defined population *with the explicit aid of a* formal randomizing device *in such a way that the* probability that any particular sample will result is specified in advance.

The terms printed in roman type above call for comment.

The Defined Population
This is sometimes a natural one ("All American women aged twenty or older"). At other times it is artificial ("All the patients considered suitable for entry in a particular randomized trial"). With the natural populations, one usually aims at descriptions, e.g.,

of prevalences, incidences, rates of inbreeding, age-structure. In artificial populations, random selection or randomization is to be done in order to study and compare the effects of experimental manipulations such as treatments. But of course the distinction is neither rigid nor absolute. For instance, some investigators who are passive (in the sense that they do not intervene) study in natural, unmanipulated, populations the relationship between smoking and lung cancer, or domicile and goiter, with the somewhat perilous goal of establishing causal relationships.

Conversely, the experimentalist, working with artificial populations, need not be quite so excruciatingly careful about the choice of his sample as the passive observer is. Any unrepresentativeness may be balanced out by randomization of his subjects into the various treatment groups. Nevertheless, while the *soundness* of the experimenter's conclusions about the manipulation may not be jeopardized by the choice of the subjects, *the scope of generalization* may be.

Example 1.2. An experiment may show beyond doubt that a drug increases growth in the legs of young male rats. If the experimenter should apply these conclusions to elderly human females, he does so at his peril. Sex hormones, for instance, may have different impacts in males and females. The drug may be highly effective in adolescence, but have no effect afterwards. Bones never seal off in rats; in human beings they do, and further growth is thereby prevented.

A simple minimum criterion of whether or not the population dealt with in a study is adequately defined is "If another investigator wished to confirm the conclusions of the study, could he with sufficient care obtain a further (separate) sample that would be comparable?" If the answer is no, then either the population is inadequately defined or the sample is idiosyncratic. These latter features do not rule out all scholarly conclusions from data of that kind. Historians often deal with the idiosyncratic and the particular; but either defect denies us any hope of nontrivial *scientific* conclusions.

Where there is, at least in principle, a defined population, it is desirable, but not absolutely necessary, that the population be explicitly numbered off. For a colony of forty experimental animals with a rare genetic trait, one may, and should, identify the subjects individually; for the human population of New York City, it may be quite impracticable to do so. Nevertheless, the population should *at the very least* be well enough defined that one could state unambiguously whether a particular person belongs to it or not.

From the standpoint of human biology, it should be possible, with sufficient resources and appropriate legal power, to construct an exhaustive list of the population (at least in principle).

Formal Randomizing Devices

Let us suppose that the objective is to construct a random sample with two properties: (*a*) each member of the population has an equal chance of being included; (*b*) all possible combinations of members that go to make up the sample (given the sample size) are equally likely. We have, at least in principle, a list of all members. At this stage an *actual, concrete, randomizing device* is used to select the sample. (Choosing them by closing one's eyes and sticking a pin in the list is an unsatisfactory device, especially if the list covers many pages.) Common useful methods are:

1. Put each name on a slip of paper of uniform size, weight, and texture, mix the slips thoroughly in an urn, and select them blind, one at a time. This method has a noble tradition, but is somewhat cumbersome for modern use on a large scale.
2. Assign a number to each subject, and use a book of random numbers to select the sample.* It is wise to pick the entry point in the table of random numbers by another randomizing device.
3. Follow the same course as in method 2, but use a mathematical device for generating the random numbers.

This phase of the process is not to be understood metaphorically. I do not mean by it that the experimenter picks the sample *as if* carrying out one of the above procedures. I mean that *he actually does carry it out faithfully as prescribed.* (The human mind is *not* an adequate randomizing device.)

The Probabilistic Properties Required of a Random Sample

The qualities required will determine, and be determined by, the pattern of random sampling. For instance, in all three methods of random selection just described, the proportion of females in the sample will be an accurate estimate of the proportion of females in the reference population. But if the sampling procedure were designed so that each unmarried man had ten times the

---

*Tables of random numbers are included in many practical textbooks on statistical method. A book by the Rand Corporation, *A Million Random Digits with 100,000 Normal Deviates* (New York: Free Press, 1955) is also available. Details on the use of random numbers are technical and are omitted here.

chance of being selected as a married man, the expected proportion of unmarried men would be a correspondingly inflated estimate of the proportion of unmarried men in the population.

There are special cases in which random sampling is done in two or more stages.

Example 1.3. We might randomly select a sample of 500 adult males in Baltimore for cardiac examination, and in turn randomly select 50 of them for echocardiography. Properly conducted, such a scheme would yield information about echocardiograms comparable to what we would have obtained by selecting 50 adult males from the population, directly and in one stage.

While this conclusion is quite sound, special conceptual problems arise when there is ambiguity as to how many sampling stages have been used. The instance just given illustrates the point. A sample picked at random from Baltimore may be seen either as representing a one-stage sample from the reference set of Baltimore, which must strictly be treated as finite and which is a statement about "people that live in Baltimore." On the other hand, it may be seen as a two-stage sample from a cosmic population, the population of Baltimore being itself seen as the sample in the first stage. The conclusions then apply to "people of the type that live in cities like Baltimore."

NONRANDOM SAMPLING

Professional laboratory scientists are, or certainly ought to be, well aware of random sampling. At times they have no need of it. For instance, nobody expects a chemist to obtain a formally random sample of molecules before exploring the properties of some chemical compound. The reasoning is that all the molecules are of the same type and are thoroughly mixed, and any usable sample contains an enormous number of them.* If need be, a population may be split up into distinct subgroups (e.g., mixtures of isotopes isolated chemically may be sorted by atomic weight; or isomers may be sorted into *d*-forms and *l*-forms) that are believed homogeneous. This subdivision, or *stratification*, may perfectly well be done after the sample is obtained. There is a somewhat dangerous tendency for biochemists to suppose that they also enjoy this exemption from random sampling conceded to the chemist: that they do not come under the canons of random sampling proper to biology.

---

*Even so, an analytical chemist quantitatively examining a crude mixture of (say) oils, would mix his sample thoroughly before taking an aliquot.

This supposition may sometimes prove sound, but is most often far from it.

To insist that clinicians use formal random sampling may be a counsel of perfection. On the one hand, too often their own approach to sampling is deplorably lax, and their sins are due to carelessness. On the other hand, their most vehement critic is apt to be "a thoughtless callow youth/Who from his books had learnt much doubtful truth." Patients do not look up a book of random numbers to see whether they should come to our clinic or not. The scientist should respect, *must* respect, the serious theories of the statistician; but Medicine is the study not merely of the ideal, the possible, and the permissible, but of the actual. If the clinic patients do not follow the rules of random sampling as laid down by the statistician, that merely tells us that those methods of the statistician cannot be used to make inferences about patients. This fact may be unpleasant, like death and taxes, but no amount of disdain will make it go away. Nothing harms the relationship between the clinician and the statistician more than superciliousness on the part of either. Little of Medicine (or of science in general) would exist, and the inspiration for practically all of public health and preventive medicine would dry up, if inferences were confined to data from random sampling (1).

Formal Warrants for Belief

Scientifically minded clinicians pride themselves on believing only adequately reasoned statements; anything less is superstition. That is a sound position. But I would make distinctions, commonly overlooked, among the several different kinds of reasons why we believe a statement. Consider three medical beliefs.

Example 1.4. Smoking increases the risk of cancer of the lung. There is as yet no altogether rational explanation for it, merely massive empirical evidence of association. Smokers have a higher incidence of lung cancer than comparable nonsmokers.

Example 1.5. There is no explanation, that I know of, why people with lung abscesses have the peculiar rounding of the fingers known as clubbing. Our firm belief in the relationship is based on the purely empirical and nonformal observations that the two are associated and that the clubbing regresses after the abscess has been adequately treated.

Example 1.6. In contrast, we have a clear, and rational, understanding of the relationship between the oxygen dissociation curve in an aberrant form of hemoglobin and the hematocrit level (i.e., the concentration of red cells in whole blood). Suppose that in a single case for a particular, newly discovered hemoglobin, it was shown that there is a high hematocrit and the hemoglobin holds on to oxygen very tightly; physicians would then accept the relationship without reserve. The onus of proof would rest firmly on any who would dispute it.

The evidential support given by random sampling is overwhelming in example 1.4, helpful and confirmatory in example 1.5, almost superfluous in example 1.6. Broadly, one should use random sampling as a means of arriving at conclusions when they are not forthcoming from other sources. What these other sources may be would call for a vast discussion of theories of knowledge. But perhaps two illustrations may help.

Example 1.7. Genetics is one of the foremost instances in biology proper of a coherent topic endowed with a coherent theory. That is, on the one hand, it has authentic structure: it deals with actually existing units, most of which have had at least some scrutiny at a physicochemical level. Genes and chromosomes are concrete. They do not have the semiabstract quality of adaptation or peripheral resistance or allergy. On the other hand, Mendelian genetics lends itself to sharp mathematical laws. Sound studies—even for pedigrees—can be performed without appeal to random sampling. That is not to say that random sampling is not useful, or even at times necessary, in genetics. But those methods based on the use of *probands* (i.e., persons in whom the disorder is first recognized in the pedigree) are commonly valid alternatives. And it is fortunate that they are, since examining the nervous system in 100,000 subjects in order to pick up one case of a lethal neurological disorder is totally impracticable, and if such a study were done the results would almost certainly not be trustworthy.* It is remarkable that geneticists are most indebted to the conventional methods of random sampling in investigating the probabilistic aspects of chromosomes, where no sound theory of behavior yet exists.

Example 1.8. Infectious disease is another field in which formal structure is invaluable. While it has a respectable mathematical theory, it is not nearly so cogent or so widely used as genetic theory is. To compensate, it has the advantage over genetics that the basic unit—the microorganism—is in many cases much more easily studied than the gene or the chromosome. It is salutary to recall how much was discovered (and is still being discovered) about the

---

*For instance, maintaining uniform diagnostic standards among the many neurologists who would be required to carry out such a gigantic study would create major problems.

natural history and the cause of infectious disease without recourse to random sampling.

I would have totally failed in my purpose if the reader were to suppose that in the foregoing section I have been decrying or belittling random sampling. My point is rather that there is often a false division of labor. There is a common (if implicit) idea that people studying populations need random sampling whereas laboratory scientists and clinicians do not. This viewpoint misses the main issue. If the clinician attempts to make inferences on the grounds that there is an *empirical* relationship, it is virtually impossible for him to escape random sampling, and he had better do it properly.

Example 1.9. At the time of writing, the association between the B27 tissue type (formerly termed W27) and ankylosing spondylitis is sound only because it is based on sound sampling (2).

Example 1.10. The demonstrated effect of sulfinpyrazone on the survivorship of blood platelets (3, 4) owes virtually nothing to random sampling.

Example 1.11. The use of short-chain fatty acids in renal disease is based on biochemical theory and (right or wrong) is a rational process. It calls for corroborative empirical studies; but it need not appeal to sampling at all.

Each type of investigator to his method. A physician floundering around with metrical definitions of disease from haphazard data (see chapter 12) is as certain to come to grief as an investigator trying to determine the pathogenesis of metachromatic leucodystrophy from questionnaires sent to millions of unselected subjects. But no good comes of seeing random and nonrandom selection as competing with one another; and there are plenty of cases where the richest yield will come from a proper attention to both.

ALTERNATIVES TO EMPIRICAL PROOF

At this point I may briefly anticipate a topic that we shall later deal with in some detail. It is that more or less adequate proof from formal evidence is not the only (and, arguably, not even the main) warrant·for our beliefs. What is acceptable to us in general is a matter not only of proof but also of plausibility. A conjecture put forward for our belief must be believable if it is to convince us. Only by the reality of this demand can one understand the perennial "obtuseness" of so many teachers in positions of influence and authority towards claims that formally had been stringently proved (for instance, the merits of antiseptic surgery, or light anesthesia in abdominal surgery). It is easy to dismiss their reluctance to believe plain evidence as inordinate conservatism. But cautious skepsis does provide a bulwark against irresponsible conjecture. Conversely, ordinate radicalism has its place; occasionally there is need for an adventurous jump outside what is known to what may be true. This kind of step ("illation") can rarely appeal to data, which do not usually exist and never will exist until the investigator takes the plunge. Rather, it stems from some idea generated by a set of facts arising in the mind of the investigator who is attempting to make sense of them. One can understand very well why this line of argument is looked on with suspicion by particular groups of scholars anxious to distinguish knowledge from fancy. But the fact that meaning does not constitute proof does not mean that it cannot, or should not, carry its own kind of conviction. No reasonable scientist will undertake a demanding line of enquiry without a strong conviction that he is on the right track. But clearly this conviction is not a matter of proof; for if the object of enquiry were already proved, the enquiry would be superfluous.

Example 1.12. Clinical investigators, quite appropriately, agonize over the controlled trial: whether they may in conscience withhold a treatment that they are sure is beneficial. But if this is not merely a way of talking and they really are sure it is beneficial, what need is there for the trial? The only sense I can make of this apparent contradiction is that proof (the trial) is not the only pathway to conviction.

PROBLEMS

1.1. At a family picnic, one of the children sees and eats a mushroom not previously known to biologists. An hour later the child develops convulsions and dies. The coroner instructing his jury suggests the following courses open to them in their findings:

    a. To declare that one can conclude nothing from one case

    b. To recommend a controlled trial on volunteers to compare the mortality rate in those who do and those who do not eat the mushroom

    c. To note that ants were seen to eat the fungus with impunity

    d. To call for expert opinions from a particle physicist and a mathematician

    e. To recommend that picnics be made illegal.

Discuss these and other options.

1.2. Identify and discuss critically the formal warrants for the following beliefs.
  a. If the arm of a human being is amputated, a new arm will never grow in its place.
  b. The earth orbits about the sun, not the converse.
  c. Derivatives of *Digitalis* are helpful in the treatment of heart failure.
  d. The physical characteristics of copper are the same everywhere in the universe and have been at all times throughout history.
  e. In any person picked at random, the number of parenchymal cells in the brain declines from the age of fifteen onward.

1.3. Consider the role (explicit or implicit) of sampling methods in the following, and consider how far violation of the rules of sampling may invalidate the conclusions.
  a. Testing the pH in a specimen of urine.
  b. Detecting a high white-cell count (leucocytosis).
  c. Obtaining a skin biopsy to study an enzyme system in cultured fibroblasts.
  d. The finding of the frequencies of blood groups in various populations that are now quoted in reference books.
  e. Justifying the orthodox view on the correct management of a Colles's fracture of the wrist.

1.4. Comment on the following titles for papers:
  a. Fatigue
  b. Chinese Influenza Complication Treatment Methods
  c. Basic Electrolyte Management
  d. A New, Probably Genetic, Syndrome of Mental Retardation, Low-set Ears, Short Stature, Dislocated Radial Heads, Scoliosis, Atrial Septal Defect, Spinal Stenosis, Peculiar Facies, Meiosis, Distichiasis, Aposiopesis, and Hendiades: Report of a Case and Review of the Literature.

1.5. Consider the following proposition: "There are two classes of patients who undergo gastrectomy: those that survive the operation and those that do not. The objective of prognosis is to distinguish between the two." In the process, *explicitly* identify *all* the assumptions made.

1.6. Christmas and the New Year are commonly thought of as seasons in which consumption of alcohol increases the risk of traffic accidents. J. A. Waller ("Holiday drinking and highway fatalities," *J Amer Med Ass* 206:2693–97, 1968) gives the data shown in the adjoining table for the number of (autopsied) deaths in car accidents in three California counties in 1960–67.

Total number of deaths during weeks		Blood alcohol in cadavers (mg/dl)	Total number of deaths during weeks	
39–50	51–52		1–13 & 39–50	51–52
1940	180	None	579	70
		1–49	38	1
		50–99	72	7
		100–149	109	3
		150–249	219	22
		250 or more	99	6

The authorities believe that special care is needed at such seasons, especially among those who have been drinking alcohol. In the light of the above data, comment critically on their beliefs.

1.7. In what way are the following methods of recruiting patients from the population likely to give unrepresentative samples?
a. Telephoning them at home
b. Telephoning them at work
c. Selecting all children attending public school and their parents
d. Random probability sampling of persons at their homes on Sundays
e. Taking every tenth visitor walking down a hospital corridor
f. Taking all blood donors.

Discuss how serious the distortion may be in typical studies of each kind.

1.8. A scholarly body organized a symposium in 1984, to which all politicians of standing were invited except for presidents, or former presidents, of the United States who are women, Black, or Jewish. Is this exclusion discriminatory?

2 | Proof and Cause

In the preceding chapter I have suggested that two of the most characteristic scientific pursuits are certainty and meaning. They are elusive, and to some extent conflicting, goals. It is easy to be certain about vague and trivial statements. Nobody disputes that the sun is hot or that jumping off cliffs is bad for the health. In contrast, the theory of evolution is an insight with gigantic meaning, but, of its nature, difficult to state scientifically. It is hard to prove even as a historical theory (which is concerned with *what* happened) and still more so as a scientific theory (which proposes to account in explicit detail for *how* it happened). We shall be returning later to this theme of the relationship between certainty and definiteness.

A further difficulty is, as it were, imposed on the ideas of proof and meaning. If we are to rest science in large part on a particular set of fundamental ideas, as a perfectly reasonable precaution we require that the ideas be submitted to the most detailed scrutiny. One would not wish to found any serious study on assumptions that contradict one another, for instance. A relentless worrying at the foundations of science raises all manner of difficulties that the lay mind does not perceive, and may have difficulty even in understanding. The mind nurtured on popular newspapers is full of glib beliefs about what science has proved concerning the cause of thunderstorms, or coronary disease, or quasars. The extent to which a scientific mind has *worried* at these fundamentals is a measure of how educated that mind is (and not merely how well processed). At heart, this concern is not *skepticism* (which is a rather morbid wallowing in doubt) but *skepsis,* which is that intellectual discipline that keeps a science honest and makes for progressive refinement in it. There is nothing in the least romantic about the proper use of scientific skepsis. It is not an assertion of *dis*belief but a continued sounding of the credentials of belief.

Example 2.1. A critic (who had supposed that some doubts of mine arose from pure timorousness or possibly even romantic skepticism) proposed as one concrete issue on which we could have no doubts, that night and day are quite different. I quibbled with this distinction: what are we to call twilight, for instance? But he argued that the indefiniteness does not lie in the notion of night and day but merely in where exactly the boundary is to be put between them. To readers who grow impatient with this discussion, I may point out that an almost exactly similar problem and discussion arise over the difference between health and disease. (We shall discuss that topic further in chapter 12.) It can be argued, indeed it is argued, that some people are incapacitated in bed with lobar pneumonia, but most people are not; and that for all practical purposes the difference is as definite as need be.

These ideas, however, are good enough only in a narrow experience; and if we try to use them without further reflection, sooner or later we will get into serious trouble. For instance, at the North Pole, what happens to our assurance that we know what "night" may be? Do we argue that even in summer there is still night for some period every twenty-four hours, but that it is a sunny night? Or that there is a night but of zero duration? Or that when we talk about "six months of night," we are not speaking in metaphors, but strictly: that north of the arctic circle we change the old definition of night from a daily to an annual cycle? Such a problem would perhaps never occur to a tropical thinker.

Likewise, to say that persons are sick *insofar as* they are incapacitated, is not foolproof either. Is pregnancy a sickness? Is old age? Is fatigue? Is grief? Because some people having early pulmonary tuberculosis can carry on without conscious disability, are we to argue that they are healthy? What are we to make of moral defects like laziness or crime or procrastination?

I do not say that these problems are insoluble. I am merely suggesting the dangers of dealing with them superficially and with insufficient thought. They become troublesome problems whenever we propose screening programs in populations, or when we try to study the genetics of disease. What is so perilous about casual common sense is that too often it involves no conscious decision at all. In the past, most physicians were not given to saying "We will agree to call it a disease if. . . ." They were not even saying "It is obvious that such and such is a disease." The difference between sickness and health seemed to them so obvious that they scarcely identified their notions as beliefs, any more than they identified the heat of the sun or the disadvantages of jumping off cliffs as beliefs. It is when one attempts *formal analysis* of the cause of disease—for instance whether or not a particular "disease" is genetic and Mendelian—that the inadequacy of casual identification of the sick becomes evident. For, often, the scientific conclusion depends on determining the frequency of a trait in a population, and the frequency turns out to depend exquisitely on just where the dividing line between the sick and the well is to be drawn.

PROOF

All in all, it is wise to abandon at the start the idea that irrefutable certainty is a reasonable goal. To be rationally certain, we would require proof. But absolutely unequivocal proof would depend on two things: on axioms that are beyond dispute and on a method of argument that is unassailable.

Axioms

As to finding indisputable axioms, there are any number of difficulties. What we accept without dispute include:

1. Disguised definitions ("All quadrupeds have four legs"), which are properly conventions or *tautologies*.
2. Matters so commonplace that we find it difficult even to identify our beliefs about them as the result of experience ("All human beings need water").
3. Things that we believe necessities of thought because we could imagine no alternative ("If George is as old as Joe, then Joe is as old as George"). Such statements tend to be either trivial or fallible, and many are both.

These three kinds of statements can be rescued by definitions. Indeed, all too often definition is used as an escape device in Medicine. Any exceptions to a rule may be disposed of by appealing to definitions and calling the exceptions something else.

Example 2.2. I can defend the claim that there exists a distinctive disease, "rheumatoid arthritis," that causes morning stiffness. Any disorder, otherwise indistinguishable, that causes no morning stiffness I may call pseudorheumatoid arthritis. There is a precedent for this specious step in the very term itself: the ending "-oid" means "having the *eidos* (or form) of;" it was originally applied to avoid confusing rheumatoid arthritis with rheumatic arthritis ("acute rheumatism"). I do not deny that the latter distinction is useful. Science is possible only because at the outset we are prepared to distinguish arbitrarily between some things and some other things. It calls for the nicest judgment as to which differences are worthy of note and which are not. But these judgments have nothing to do with proof except that, if abused, they tend to lead either to absurdities or to trivialities in proof.

Axioms that embody nothing more than common experience (which is always finite, and hence almost always incomplete) are perpetually at the mercy of some rare exception (which is apt to be labeled "miraculous"); or they may be destroyed by some unforeseen structural anomaly in the notions underlying it. (One cannot argue from both the axiom "Health must be promoted at any cost" and "The budget for health must be kept within inexorable limits.")

Example 2.3. Take the famous riddle posed by Lewis Carroll. The axiom is the particular, and innocent-looking, statement that the (male) village barber shaves every male in the village who does not shave himself. Does he shave himself or not? Either answer means that the axiom is violated. The same paradox is met in a book that lists all the books that are not listed in a book. Does it contain its own name or not? The cause of the paradox is ultimately that in each case we are trying to make one member of a symmetrical class into a privileged member, having a unique relationship to the class as a whole. The mathematician Russell would have said that the fault stems from mixing languages of different orders (5).

Example 2.4. The reader who supposes at this stage that I have wandered off into amusing, but irrelevant, asides would do well to think of how one might set limits for sanity. The difficulties are twofold. First we have no *natural, objective, quantitative* scales on which we can measure the intellectual, behavioral, moral, and emotional aspects of the mind, the factors ordinarily assessed in deciding sanity. Measurements do exist (for instance, intelligence tests) but, however well entrenched, they are still arbitrary. They have been devised by human beings in historic time on the basis of what they themselves have seen as normal. They have been tried out on samples that are not necessarily representative of the human race. The other problem is that, in something so ultimately human as the mind and its contents, we become involved inescapably in value judgments. In principle, the physicist may soundly and accurately measure the weight of a man without getting involved in the question of whether that is a good weight or whether some other one would be preferable. But one might then ask, Why should the *clinician* make the measurement unless something of importance depends on it? In the same fashion the psychometrician by his *selection* of tests (however well standardized and reproducible they are) implies an importance in the things that he chooses; and this criticism is important in itself even without getting into the problem of how he is to score the results.

Despite these defects, some may have no misgivings about any actual dangers. But a hostile adversary could point out causes for concern. First, psychiatrists are not themselves altogether immune to the diseases in which they themselves deal. No doubt there are excellent reasons for that fact. One is occupational exposure. Pathologists know more about disease than most physicians; but the rate of hepatitis among them is higher. For the psychiatrist to listen many hours a day to patients' gloom must itself be gloomy. Some few psychiatrists may have injudiciously adopted their profession precisely because they were themselves in need of psychiatric help. (Indeed, part of the psychoanalytic training is to go through a full psychoanalysis.) The many psychiatrists I have known have been eminently sane people. Those few that will in due course get into trouble are not the normal ones. Yet even they may be making decisions about the sanity of some patients, just as there are doubtless mad surgeons or judges or airline pilots in whose hands the lives of people are entrusted. The safeguards are not only that all these people are themselves monitored but that there is enough redundancy in the system (a resident clinical staff, a court of appeals, a copilot) to provide security. But redundancy is no safeguard against collective delusion.

Example 2.5. In a notorious study (6) it was shown that some observers who, to test the system, simulated insanity and were committed to mental institutions found it excessively difficult to get discharged when they confessed their deceit. That study may mean many things. (Readers might with benefit stop and think about it before reading further. It will reveal something of their own prejudices as well as their insights.) It may mean that psychiatrists are prejudiced against supposing the sanity of their patients. It may mean that the desire to simulate madness is seen by the psychiatrist as a form of madness.* It may mean that by being in a mental hospital, even sane people, unwittingly imitate the telltale marks of the insane. It may be that the volunteers were not, in fact, sane. It

---

*It is consonant with the famous Goldwynism: "Anybody who goes to a psychiatrist should have his head examined."

may mean that they were out to make a point, and that even when confessing the hoax, they were not playing fair with the psychiatrist. But the example raises at least misgivings that there do not, in fact, exist secure ways of telling the insane from the malingerer.†

The problem is wider still. Who is to say when those at odds with society are the authentic visionaries, artists, scientists, geniuses, and when they are mad or bad, psychopaths, fakes, and the rest? I have no solution to propose; nor do I wish to convey an exaggerated sense of an impending disaster that my unanswered question bespeaks. We must make practical decisions and trust in them without being uncritical. But these problems are by no means trivial: I would counsel particularly against falsely allaying anxiety by the common experience that most problems solve themselves without need of much finesse. The fact that most of the time these misgivings are of only theoretical importance does not mean that they are imaginary or guarantee that they will never prove to be catastrophic. Two particular areas for concern are at the interface with other disciplines (notably law, politics, and theology) and wherever one is extrapolating beyond actual experience.

The Methods of Argument

Once the problems of axioms have been dealt with, we are concerned with two issues.

The first is a rather theoretical issue. How, in general, do we defend a particular method of proof? Several methods exist that we shall review in due course: deductive, inductive (in both the logical and the mathematical senses), deductive testing, stochastic proof, etc. Clearly the defence of methods of proof cannot itself be a proof. One cannot prove the validity of deductive proof in general by means of deductive proofs or by using inductive proof which is then validated by deductive proofs. Sooner or later one has to appeal to native common sense, which will balk at conclusions that are utterly repugnant or that lead to irreconcilable paradoxes. It may come as a surprise to some that a proof may be overthrown by empirical experience. Some examples are obvious (e.g., one can readily demolish the proof that bees cannot fly).

Example 2.6. In a famous instance a distinguished statistical theo-

---

†This example must not be construed as an attack on the competence of psychiatrists. Far from it. To note that sometimes a surgical operation causes shock that kills a patient is not an attack on surgeons. The point is that psychiatrists and surgeons, by their very natures, deal with balancing deliberately calculated risks. Rosenhan's thoughtful sequel (7) has some important ideas to communicate.

rist Karl Pearson (8) gave an incorrect formula for interpreting a statistical procedure, known as the chi-square test. The actual details of what the test means or what Pearson's fallacy was* are quite beside the point here. It is of interest that the error was first discovered (9) by those who found that there were too few false "significant" results. The error that Pearson had made was subsequently remedied by another theorist, R. A. Fisher (10).

The second group of problems in proof revolve around technical competence. There are rules to be obeyed if a proof is to be a sound one.

Deductive Proof. Deductive proof is well known and is described in the standard textbooks. The method used is to argue from generally applicable axioms to particular cases or classes of cases. In science it works admirably when the axioms are well-established (for instance in Mendelian genetics). Its main medical scope is in the application of principles rather than in their discovery. It has little enough usefulness in biological science, although I have found that it furnishes a valuable analogy in scientific exploration of cause (11).

Inductive Proof. This method argues from a (necessarily limited) number of experiences to a general truth. As a general means of rigorous proof, it runs into insurmountable difficulties that were exposed in the eighteenth century. Induction of this type is best seen as a source of inspiration for conjecture rather than as definitive proof.

Example 2.7. The human chromosomes are given conventional numbers, the largest pairs having the lowest numbers. The fact that in living populations human subjects do not occur in whom one of the pair of autosomes number 1 is missing suggests that the absence of this chromosome is incompatible with life. But this argument is not the same as proof by experimental intervention.

It is common wisdom that the larger our pertinent experience of a principle to which there are no exceptions, the more sure we are that the generalization is sound. Statistics deals with the question of how sure we are entitled to be. Nevertheless, any claims that the principle is universally true would be demolished by even one counterexample, however long it was in coming. Thus, our accumulated experience can never constitute unassailable proof. This residual uncertainty, from which we scientists never entirely escape, is healthy. It helps us to keep our minds open; but farfetched

---

*He gave the wrong rule for calculating the degrees of freedom.

theoretical possibilities should never be used as a warrant for endless neurotic vacillation in dealing with practical issues that call for prompt decisions.

One must be careful in using general experience to overtrump the evidence in the particular case. There is an important (and I suspect irreconcilable) difference between making clinical decisions and assembling scientific facts. But the difference is easily overlooked and may lead to false conclusions.

Example 2.8. Headache is a rare manifestation of multiple sclerosis, a diagnosis that the neurologist would be very reluctant to invoke to explain it. In arriving at the best diagnosis for a particular patient, it is right and proper for the clinician to use this fact. But the resulting *diagnostic decision* is not a scientific datum. One may not use the diagnosis made in the patient to throw any light on the relationship between headache and multiple sclerosis, precisely because the headache is used (if only as contributory evidence) to make the diagnosis. One may not appeal to the relationship to make the individual diagnosis and then use the fact that the finding is present in the patient so diagnosed to prove that the appeal was legitimate.

This kind of circular argument is a common one: not only in Medicine but in science generally. It is surprising how many professional people are prepared to declare something almost impossible on the grounds that it has hardly ever been previously described. It is easily shown (12) that if this line of argument is used to build up one's experience, it tends to give an estimate of the frequency that is something close to the square of the true frequency. For a rare trait, the estimate will be much too low.

Mathematical Induction. There is another use of the term *inductive proof* in mathematics that is quite different in character and is accepted as rigorous. The argument is of the form: If the fact that a proposition is true for any case in a sequence means that it is therefore true for the consecutive case, then if it is true for the first, it is true for all.

Example 2.9. So far, the oldest known survivor with Hurler syndrome has died before the age of twenty-five. Thus, the second longest-lived died even earlier, and therefore before the age twenty-five; and hence, by mathematical induction, all cases died before twenty-five. (The argument is trivial and labored, but valid.)

Proof by Analogy. This method often enjoys great flexibility and furnishes much insight. Purely symbolic proofs (i.e., those based on manipulating mathematical symbols in accordance with a special type of algebra) are subtle and agile; the greatest weakness in their application is irrelevancy.

• *The soundness of an analogy depends on how faithfully the terms of the discussion are translated into symbols, and how faithfully the conclusion from the manipulation of the symbols is translated back.*

Thus, many words are ambiguous—*pain, responsible, fitness,* for instance—and one must be careful not to get their various meanings confused in the process of translation. For my part, I see proofs by analogy as suggestive but, in the biological fields, rarely compelling.

Example 2.10. It may be useful in some ways to see a perforated bowel as like a burst pipe. But it would be deplorable to see it in these terms alone. Surgical problems must be solved inside the context of surgery (with due attention to shock, infection, and tissue reaction) and not exclusively by an appeal to plumbing.

I fancy that the guiding principles of medical conduct are in such a primitive state because those relatively few writers that have attempted a systematic analysis of the problems have relied far too heavily on rather inadequate analogies with other fields. There is another defect in so many of our medical proofs—a quite inadequate analysis and characterization of our terms—that I shall defer for fuller treatment until the third section of this book.

Two popular forms of proof widely used in medicine may also be mentioned.

Proof by Exclusion

Example 2.11. In a medical chart, one may find a note such as "Rule out subacute combined degeneration of the cord." The intent might be put somewhat as follows. "This diagnosis is here implausible, but the disease, though devastating, is readily treatable with high success; and it would be a major mistake to fail to recognize it, in however atypical a form. Hence, we will do special tests for it, but with little hope that they will be positive." As far as it goes, this argument is admirable Medicine.

But what if, on the balance of the evidence, but still incorrectly, we do rule it out? It is largely a myth that one can exclude some diseases as impossibilities and that by default the diagnosis *must* be something else. Unfortunately, a spurious reassurance is commonly given by talking about "primary," "essential," "idiopathic," and "agnogenic" diseases, by the use of words ending in "-osis" and "-opathy," and by almost any diagnosis exceeding fifteen letters in length.

Example 2.12. If I have tried to find a cause for somebody's high blood pressure, having worked my way down a list of some thirty possibilities and drawn a blank with each, the proper stance is simply to say I do not know. To call it "essential hypertension" contributes nothing but obscuration to the simple fact of my ignorance. The argument that in most instances of high blood pressure no definable cause is known and that we are going to have to admit our ignorance embarrassingly often leaves me quite unmoved.

Example 2.13. Likewise, in some cases a genetic disease is not due to a single gene or to a chromosomal abnormality. I gain nothing whatsoever by crowding the remaining collection of genetic diseases under an umbrella term "multifactorial" (or in Greek, "polygenic"). Not only is this a structureless notion* but it may convey a kind of spurious definiteness in the minds of those who use the term.

But a far greater problem with proofs by exclusion is that, in practice, they rarely exclude. A theoretically perfect way of doing so would be to make an exhaustive list, *prove* it is exhaustive, and demolish all but one possibility. The most difficult step is the second; it is usually not easy to see how we can prove that the list is exhaustive. In practice, many clinicians would work with a list of every possibility they could think of; and how many gaps there are in it is some measure of their knowledge and judgment. To assert that some particular diagnosis must be correct *because one cannot think of any other possibility* is, to say the least, precarious, and occasionally disastrous.

Example 2.14. A good psychiatrist will never let the diagnosis of hysteria be made by exclusion alone. To exclude 95 percent of the possibilities still leaves 5 percent, which, while small, may still be much greater than the frequency of the disease being diagnosed by exclusion. This cautionary thought leads to my last type of proof.

Stochastic Proof. In my view the usual (perhaps the universal) type of proof in medicine involves judgment. *Stochastic* originally meant "guessing"; it now means much the same as "probabilistic." In such proofs one abandons all pretensions to certainty, recognizing that there are few signs in medicine that unequivocally either establish or demolish a diagnosis. (It is said that the Argyll-Robertson pupil occurs only in quaternary syphilis; that posttussive suction occurs only in cavitation of the lung. I cannot vouch for any of such claims.)

Example 2.15. It is common teaching that the rare X-linked disorder incontinentia pigmenti never occurs in males. There is a common, and I suspect prudent, dictum: Never say "never" in

---

*In contrast, the term *Galtonian* has a well-defined structure. However, it by no means exhausts the patterns not included in the Mendelian or chromosomal groups (13), and hence is not arrived at merely by exclusion. We shall have a good deal more to say about this topic in chapter 12.

medicine. Most universals are sustained artificially. If what looks like incontinentia pigmenti occurs in a male, it is perhaps called Naegeli's syndrome (14).

The idea of stochastic proof (which will be more fully developed in chapter 6) is that taking both the frequency and the features of a disease into account, one can state the relative odds that a patient has disease A and disease B. If no decision hangs on the diagnosis, one may leave it at that. If one *must* make a decision, e.g., to operate or not, the best decision will certainly involve more than mere odds: for instance, the several costs of possible incorrect courses of action.

But there are three points that merit special attention before I leave the topic for the time being.

First, even to do nothing is a course of action.

Second, there is no such thing as playing it safe. This expression usually means putting undue emphasis on one side of the argument. My objective would be, not to avoid one type of mistake altogether, but to minimize the total errors of all types and the damage they might do. That is, I do not play it safe, I play it safest.

Third, some decisions (e.g., an amputation) are irrevocable; others (e.g., many medical treatments) are not. Where a revocable treatment is given over time, the effects (good or bad) of the treatment will give evidence as to whether the treatment should be stopped, continued, or intensified. A colleague once took me severely to task for discussing diagnosis, prognosis, and treatment as if they were totally separable processes. He is, of course, quite right. It is asking for trouble ever to let authentic medicine become the slave of our abstractions.

Proof by Congeries. One is so accustomed to the rather artificial way that the history of science is presented (especially by the amateur historian) that it is not easy to grasp or describe how discoveries are actually made. Rigorous proofs are a large part of the ideals of formal science; but too often they are the enemies of discovery, which, as much as anything else, is an imaginative process. Here one has to be cautious. To say that a narrow focus on proof is stultifying is not to glorify grandiose speculation.

However, there are many instances in which formal proof is not possible, and yet a great many loose proofs, no one of which would bear close scrutiny, are highly convincing in aggregate. The image this method suggests is a group of men trying to find their way, one of whom cannot see, one who cannot walk, one who can read the names of the streets but does not understand maps, and so on. In effect, they succeed collectively by complementing each other.

Example 2.16. Commonly, Harvey's discovery of the circulation (1628) is presented as if he had inherited confusion and replaced it by a theory that he proved beyond dispute. But that is not true: one of the awkward suppositions his predecessors had been forced to make in their ebb and flow theory was that blood gets from the pulmonary to the systemic vessels through pores in the cardiac septa, pores so small that nobody could find them. Harvey was forced to conclude that the exchange occurs, not there, but at the ends of the arteries and the veins through openings so small that nobody could demonstrate them either. Harvey's theory was literally full of holes. It was not until 1661 that Malpighi demonstrated the capillary bed by microscopy.* Much of Harvey's proof was circumstantial; and indeed, it is only with the introduction of contrast methods that the claim for Harvey's theory of circulation can be said to have been fully sustained.

CAUSE

At one level, cause is an easy topic to discuss: much of what we have said about giving a proof can, with a little ingenuity, be adapted to enquiry into cause. The difficulties lie in the old familiar area. How are we to set up a correspondence between the formal study of cause and the concrete notions of the empirical world?

For instance, we commonly think in terms as discrete as billiard balls. Smoking (one thing, a cause) causes lung cancer (another thing, an effect). In turn, lung cancer (now a cause) leads to hemoptysis (another thing, an effect). Hemoptysis (a cause) produces anemia. Anemia causes fatigue. And so forth. What do we mean by saying that smoking is a cause and lung cancer an effect? One pragmatic answer is that we can manipulate smoking (e.g., by banning it even partially) and, without affecting the lungs through any other mechanism, can thereby reduce lung cancer.

Now that kind of notion, though not infallible (as we shall see) is useful up to a point. When we examine it more closely, however, we find that there are some rather important ideas and assumptions that need to be brought out into the open and looked at carefully. For instance, it implies that what happens can be divided

---

*L. G. Wilson ("The transformation of ancient concepts of respiration in the seventeenth century," *Isis* 51:161–72, 1960) regards the earliest anatomical description of the capillary network to be Malpighi's letter *Duae epistolae de pulmonibus* (Florence, 1661). I am grateful to Dr. D. F. Proctor for guidance and helpful discussion on this point.

into units; that we can manipulate the units individually; that we know how they would have behaved if we had not manipulated them; that we have a criterion by which we can identify an authentic change. These may or may not be obvious in smoking and lung cancer; but we will not always find them simple to apply.

Discreteness

For instance, much of the teaching about standards of behavior in medicine makes constant appeal to the notion that there are discrete chunks of matter ("things"), of form ("states"), of activity ("acts"). Is it proper for a surgeon to do an operation to cure a sick person even if it endangers the life of another?

Example 2.17. A classical quandary for the gynecologist is removing a fibroid from a pregnant uterus. The terms of the question imply that the mother and fetus are distinct individuals ("things"); that a fibroid is a condition of uterine tissue sufficiently definite that we can define it as a diseased state; and that the operation is a single, homogeneous act without parts, which must needs be judged only in its entirety.

These may be perfectly reasonable suppositions in this particular case; but they must be systematically explored and sustained in all examples* if the whole field is to be put on a sound basis. It is not difficult to think of analogous situations that are much more ambiguous. Are Siamese twins one person? Or two? Or sometimes one and sometimes two? If so, how do we decide? Is old age a disease? If so, when does it start? Does it become more of a disease if we translate it into Latin and call it "senility"? Can we warrant cosmetic surgery on the grounds that ugliness is a disease? If a plastic surgeon does a sequence of ten operations to repair a facial defect, is each operation a single act, or does the whole series constitute a single act? Is the management of (say) a diabetic coma by a continuous intravenous infusion and repeated injections a single act? If this treatment is given against a patient's express wishes, it is assault and battery. But is each injection then a separate crime or all part of one crime? Is the education of a child, or a psychoanalysis, a single act?

These issues are not mere quibbles. In my view, our guidelines

---

*I obviously do not mean that conceivable cases must be exhaustively dealt with before we can establish a working principle. But it remains a working principle, not an inalienable truth; and at the mercy of any future exception. That is, it must always be a provisional principle to which one may not rationally give altogether unqualified assent.

for medical conduct are in so confused a state because of a failure to address questions of this kind. Whether one is going to argue in terms of things that behave like billiard balls or otherwise is surely a fundamental issue that should be addressed at the start and not be repeatedly stumbled over as each new problem arises. For a formal theory of appropriate action is not a featureless catalogue of recipes compiled out of thin air for use in an inexhaustible list of individual cases. Individual experience does not qualify as a coherent theory any more than a judge's sorting out the particular facts in a trial for slander is jurisprudence.

All these familiar problems should carry over into scientific enquiry. Science demands generalization: it cannot merely be an infinite bill of particulars. So it must have some shape or structure inside which we can argue; and the less forced this structure, the more adaptable and durable it will prove. Consider this macabre comment about jumping off a cliff: "It is not the jump that kills you, but the sudden stop at the end of it." Does it not shock because it implies that we are to see the flight and the impact as separable?

Example 2.18. What do we imply by saying that coronary thrombosis causes myocardial infarction? As far as it goes, the statement has merit. But one should not see the thrombosis as the villain of the piece. The final act of occlusion (i.e., blocking off of the artery) is not *ideally* to be prevented by abolishing coagulation and paralyzing platelet aggregation. Natural processes for doing so already exist. If they did not, the person would never have lived long enough to develop coronary disease. There can be no reasonable doubt that, at least sometimes, the "atheroma," the disfiguration of the arterial wall, is not merely the factor that precipitates the thrombosis but is itself the end result of a previous thrombosis. The first, unobtrusive, step in the whole process may occur very early in life (15). If scarring and thrombosis alternate, each aggravating each, it seems to be of little use to haggle over which is the cause and which the effect.

Example 2.19. In the same way, if emotional estrangement leads to behavioral upset which, in turn, leads to further estrangement, what good is it after the event to argue over which is the hen and which the egg?

The concern in both instances is that—by whatever subtle quantitative disturbances—the patient is disabled. Our way of handling that kind of upset effectively may consist of arbitrarily, even artificially, breaking a complicated, and not necessarily discrete, succession of activities; and success may tell us nothing at all about billiard-ball causality.

All I can hope to do here is to awaken some sense of the peril of shallow and mechanical arguments; and my aim is to preserve both a practical sense and a critical insight.

Example 2.20. Streptococcal sore throats should undoubtedly be treated by antibiotics. But it would be bad medicine to suppose that the cause of the disease is nothing more than the presence of the organisms. Alert clinicians know that the organisms are widespread in nature. They will wonder (in the patient with recurrent throat infections at least) about causal contributions from mechanical or immunological disorders, patterns of behavior, occupation, and so forth.

Manipulation

The theory of experiments largely depends on the notion that subjects may be randomly allocated ("randomized") to groups that are then given different treatments. The results are then compared. This practice involves a technical use of manipulation, of something that is outside the system under study (11). Manipulation has two features: its form may be inferred from what follows it; it cannot be inferred from what went on before it. We suppose that the differing consequences to the various treatment groups in a properly designed experiment are due to the manipulations that are said to be their cause. But theory demands that how the assignments to experimental groups are to be made shall not depend on the system. The whole pattern means that the manipulation is related to the system in its effect, but not in its cause. Some examples may help to make this elusive idea clearer.

Example 2.21. Lightning precedes thunder; but we do not for that reason conclude that it *causes* thunder, since lightning is not a manipulation, but is itself part of whatever it is that causes the thunder.

Example 2.22. The act of volunteering to participate in an experiment cannot safely be seen as a manipulation. Volunteers are not a random selection from the population, for example. Not only may they be highly atypical, but their decision to participate may have been influenced by the design of the experiment, which may offer payment, medical care, food supplements, or other perquisites. If volunteers do well on treatment with a drug, it may not be due to the effect of the drug itself (which may be inert); instead, it may be due to the suggestible personalities of volunteers, or to the secondary physical benefits derived at the same time.

The only way one can infer from such subjects whether the drug has this effect is to assign them to treatments (placebo or one level—or perhaps several different levels—of dosage) in a fashion that is independent of all those other factors that may influence the outcome. But in general we do not know *all* the pertinent factors. There may be unidentified genetic factors or acquired allergies or psychological components. So we get around the logical problem by making the assignment random, and then in analyzing the results, we capitalize on the fact that they have been randomized. Of course, for any particular sample we do not imagine that the various groups will be exactly equal in all respects; but at least we eliminate biases, that is, *systematic* inequalities (see chapter 3); and the analysis will take into account, and interpret, the random fluctuations in the actual outcome. Even with random assignment, one is wise to confine strict conclusions from studies on volunteers to statements about subjects who volunteer on the same terms.

Example 2.23. A study on volunteers on the use of dental floss in preventing dental caries needs to take into account the possibility that the volunteers may be those most concerned about their teeth and already using fluoride regularly. Dental floss may have an effect only when fluoride is being applied.

Example 2.24. Obviously treatment-to-effect (e.g., treatment of diabetics by dosage that is in any way influenced by the response to previous doses) cannot be seen as a manipulation, and interpretation of data from such a process gives rise to complicated logical problems.

Indeterminacy

There is a deeper demand, however. I cannot personally make any sense of the idea of a manipulation in a strictly deterministic world, i.e., one in which every event has a cause and there is no slack that cannot, at least in principle, be accounted for. On the one hand, if the behavior of each state is rigidly determined by its antecedents, I do not see on what rational grounds we can separate the whole system into component parts: how we could escape the idea that all of history is one event about one thing (11). But even setting that issue aside, the notion of a manipulation that is at once minutely determined by its antecedents and yet totally independent of them is beyond my capacity for resolving paradoxes. On these terms, I can see no difference at all between passive, i.e., unmanipulative, observation (such as the astronomer or the archeologist makes) and experimental studies. The problems of bias and confounding, which I shall deal with in chapter 3, and which are classical pitfalls of inference, seem to me quite meaningless unless there is in principle some way of authentically separating components within the system. I shall address this problem of indeterminacy in greater detail in chapter 8.

Preventive Medicine

Preventive medicine—the study of the methods of anticipating disease—points out that many of these issues are by no means academic. The kinds of data bearing on diagnosis and assessment of prevention have a notoriously ambiguous character. A sign or measurement may be a cause of the disease, or an early sign of a destined disease, or a sign that the disease is already there but not yet overt.

Example 2.25. A *known* exposure to inorganic lead is a cause of lead poisoning.

Example 2.26. Evidence that a pertinent gene has been inherited (perhaps evidence obtained by examining the gene itself) may well show that the person is destined to develop an age-dependent disorder, such as familial polyposis coli or Huntington's disease, at a stage at which the most careful *clinical* examination shows no abnormality.

Example 2.27. Electrocardiographic abnormalities may show that subclinical coronary disease is already present.

It is often difficult to say to which of these categories a finding belongs. Such ambiguity has two important consequences.

First, it bears on what is to be expected from clinical management.

Example 2.28. Classical signs of cavitation of a lung mean that one cannot anticipate the cavitation, merely try to heal it and to prevent it from extending.

Example 2.29. Evidence that lead is accumulating in the body of a person who has no signs or symptoms means that proper handling will head off the latter.

Example 2.30. A baby deficient in the enzyme galactose-1-phosphate uridyl transferase may be saved from the serious effects of galactosemia by proper and prompt dietary management from the moment of birth.

Second, there is a distinction commonly made between primary and secondary prevention: that is, between preventing the disease in the first place (e.g., environmental control of toxins) and secondary prevention that aims to forestall recurrence or further complications (e.g., orthopedic treatment of bowing of the legs to prevent osteoarthritis in the knees and to restore normal distribution of stresses at the hip and ankle). The more radical ambitions of preventive medicine are directed towards primary prevention, such as the use of immunization against poliomyelitis rather than rehabilitation of those that have recovered from it. But it seems clear enough that unless it is known how and where the measure is acting, one may easily have false confidence in the measures available. It is too easy to suppose that prevention is primary when it is secondary.

Example 2.31. I mentioned above that the earliest events in atherosclerosis may occur very early in life, so that most of the preventive measures are, in fact, secondary. The statement would doubtless be disputed. The evidence I would cite would include, for instance, the facts that one can show that already the flow patterns around orifices and the small deposits that occur nearby correspond to the lesions that occur in atherosclerosis. But in tracing back the origins of disease, there must come a point at which one has to address the cardinal problem of when the disease can be said to be present and when the normal has not been transgressed. Even at this stage it will be obvious that one can make secondary prevention look like primary by insisting on stringent (and therefore more advanced) evidence of disease, and conversely. For my part, I do not think that this kind of dispute is profitable, since it usually comes down to disputes about how words ought to be used.

Example 2.32. Primary prevention of familial polyposis coli might be construed to mean regular clinical examination to discover polyps early, or colectomy at birth, or directive genetic counseling, or removal of environmental mutagens that gave rise to the original gene, or changing something that operates even earlier than that. I suggest that the real issue is not what we call the policy but what its impact may be in the domain of human fulfillment. That is a difficult question to answer satisfactorily; but the answer is not to be found by shallow manipulations of slogans.

PROBLEMS

2.1. Consider the problems of determining on what grounds eugenic policy should be decided.

2.2. The beautiful baby contests of the twenties put a good deal of emphasis on "nourishment" (i.e., plumpness). Do you think that this fact may have had any impact on the peak wave of coronary disease in the sixties? If it did, would you draw any general conclusions that would make for future cautions in coronary disease and other fields?

2.3. Discuss constructively the role in modern medicine of diagnosing fits due to *etc.* ("idiopathic epilepsy"), scaly patches of skin that look like smallpox ("pityriasis lichenoides et varioliformis"), and the shaking palsy without the shakes ("paralysis agitans sine agitatione").

2.4. Systematically construct a list of causes of breathlessness, and prove that it is exhaustive.

2.5. Discuss how one might explore the thesis "All violent criminals are sick."

2.6. Compare closely the natures of the following statements.
   a. Scurvy is due to a deficiency of vitamin C.
   b. 5 percent of all Americans are mentally backward.
   c. The hardness of bone is due to its ability to resist deformation.

2.7. Consider whether the following are genetic or environmental:
   a. Sunburn
   b. Scurvy
   c. Child abuse
   d. Eidetic imagery ("photographic memory")
   e. Ugliness.

2.8. Veatch (16) in an interesting textbook addresses the issue of informed consent. His test case (chosen, I imagine, because it is trivial and unclouded by issues other than formal consent) deals with whether the mother's permission should be sought to obtain a specimen from the placenta of her newborn child. Analyze the biological issues. (Hint: Whose tissue is it?)

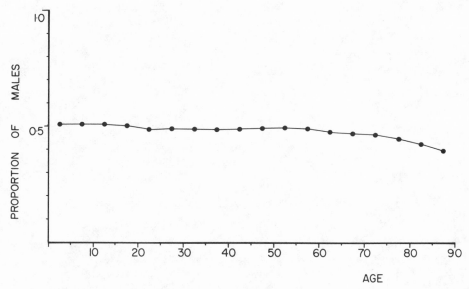

Figure 2.1. The influence of age on the sex of a person.
Source: Census of Population 1960, vol. 1, part 1, table 45.

2.9. Figure 2,1 shows the proportion of males in the American population (as determined in the 1960 census) as a function of age. We conclude that after their mid-forties, about one-fifth of all men turn into women. Critically examine the foregoing argument with an eye to avoiding a whole class of similar fallacies.

3 | Bias, Confounding, and Ambiguity

As we have seen, when we look for the cause of a disease or of some smaller anomaly in man, most often it is hard to find simple answers. The wisdom from the past tells us to study each of the likely causes by manipulating them one at a time. But there are two snags. First, there is usually no method by which we can take the whole nest of causes apart so that we may study each by itself. We cannot isolate the heart of a human being in such a way as to keep out the effects of the sympathetic nerves, the lungs and other neighboring organs, and so forth. If nothing else, there are moral and legal reasons for not doing such a study. But second, even if we could do studies of this kind without fear or hindrance, it is not at all sure that we should be much closer to understanding.

While much of modern science is based on the idea that there is nothing more to a system than its parts, there is a perceptible countertrend to this view. After having heard each musician play alone, an experienced conductor might perhaps be able to predict how they would perform together as an orchestra; but at the very least, the skill to do so is not readily learnt. (Those who can take this step commonly speak of their intuitions. Perhaps the difficulty is merely a matter of complexity; but it is also possible that properties become evident when the whole is put together that (at least, without much experience) could not be guessed however well one knows the parts. The players, for instance, would listen, and respond, to each other. It is not hard to find cases where the outcome is counterintuitive—that is, at odds with what one might guess would happen.)

Example 3.1. It seems implausible, that, other things being equal, a positive history of an inherited disease among members of the

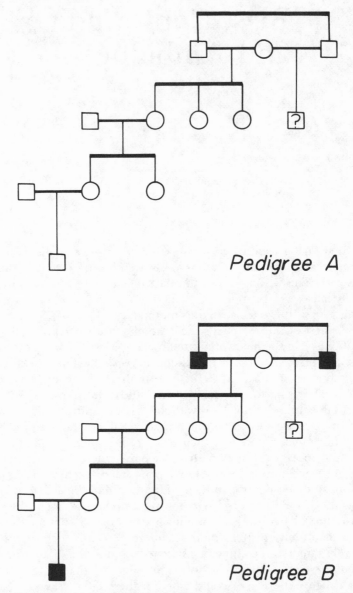

Pedigree A

Pedigree B

Figure 3.1. A paradox of family history. These pedigrees are identical in all respects except that in pedigree *B* three of the males (*square symbols*) are affected by an X-linked condition. In pedigree *A*, despite the lack of family history of the disease, the risk to the male marked by the question mark is somewhat greater than for his counterpart in pedigree *B*.

family makes the diagnosis of that disease in a specified patient *less* likely than if there is no such history. But it can be shown not only that this odd fact may be true but that this paradoxical result can be readily deduced from Mendel's laws. (See fig. 3.1.)

Likewise, one can set up a genetic system with two loci and two pairs of genes, of which one, though in itself lethal, does not die out but becomes universal (17). Or again, one may show that early diagnosis and treatment of certain cancers, especially heterogeneous ones, may lead to a higher death rate. If the diagnosis is made early, it will include many of the most severely affected patients, who would not live long enough to be included in the later study. In the same way, the expectation of life decreases with age; but the expectation of life in newborn infants is less than it is in those one year old.

Such instances (of which there are many) should, if nothing else, make us somewhat cautious about guessing how the whole behaves from what we know about the behavior of the parts. We cannot afford to make naive inferences about what goes on from casual studies. When a treatment is given to a patient, the change that we see following it is the combined effect ("the algebraic resultant") of an unknown number of individual effects.

Example 3.2. What, for instance, does lowering the blood pressure do to angina pectoris?* On the one hand, it lowers the load of work that the heart has to do, which will tend to relieve the pain; on the other hand, it lowers the pressure that feeds blood into the coronary arteries, which tends to aggravate the disorder. It is not at once obvious which effect will be the greater; and most often the answer must be found in the particular patient by trying it out.

Thus, at the least, we must give some thought to systems that are not altogether simple; and while it would be too big a task to deal with the problem in its entirety, we may make bold to deal with a few of the simpler systems.

BIAS

In many fields, most of what we know comes from sorting data into categories and finding the proportion that fall into each. We find the prevalence of multiple sclerosis, a chronic disease of the

---

Angina pectoris is a term used of a peculiar kind of pain that occurs in the chest when the load of work on the heart is increased by physical exercise, emotion, etc. It is ascribed to blood flow through the coronary arteries (the blood vessels feeding the muscle of the heart itself) being inadequate to meet the oxygen needs of the heart.

nervous system, by examining members from a sample and deciding how many of them have the disease. The prevalence is expressed as a ratio, or as that ratio multiplied by some number and
expressed as so many cases per hundred, or per thousand, or per
million. Now the sample value for such a ratio (even if it is of only
modest usefulness) can, and ideally should, be accurate in what it
aims to say. Of course, if the sample is small, we cannot hope that
the ratio we get will always be precise,* that is, near to the average
value, because (as we shall see in the second part of this book) the
effects of chance are biggest when the samples are small. But while
this random part of the error is most obtrusive for small sizes of the
sample, a big sample need not give the right answer either; too
often we find that it is flawed by what is called bias (11).

DEFINITION. Bias *is any trend in the choice of a sample, the making of
measurements on it, the analysis or publication of the findings, that tends
to give or communicate an answer that differs systematically (nonran-
domly) from the true answer.*

Note, first, that we suppose that a random sample (of the kind
we discussed in the first chapter) is being taken. In this step we
have to be careful about two main types of mistake. The first is that
the sampling procedure may be improper. The second is that the
reference population is unclear. Let us take the two points in turn.

The Sampling Procedure
    In the first chapter we met briefly the special method of pro-
bands, a way of finding groups of cases of a disease, usually a rare
one. The method fastens on to the fact that cases collected by this
means are not independent, and if there is some precise theory as
to how they are mutually dependent, it may be tested or, if it is
already established, it may be used to estimate certain quantities.
However, any sound sampling procedure must conform to the
assumptions underlying the theory.
    Example 3.3. One area of special interest to me has been familial
polyposis of the colon (18). Characteristically, the polyps are multiple, but the individual polyp is in no way distinguishable from
polyps in people who do not have this heritable disorder; and since
the condition is moderately rare and the diagnosis apt to be made
by accident, it seems reasonable in analysis to make use of a method
of probands. However, part of the diagnosis is to decide that the

---

*The distinction between precision and accuracy will be made much clearer in
chapter 10.

condition is familial, and the natural criterion is to see whether there is another affected person in the pedigree. But if we invoke this criterion, clearly we will not identify those hereditary cases in which, by chance, only one person (the proband) is affected. In effect, we must have two probands in a family to show that it is familial. This demand is not at all unreasonable; but it should be taken into account in the analysis.

Example 3.4. In contrast, the suspicion that a person with polyposis coli may have one particular kind of heritable type, the Gardner syndrome, will be made highly probable if there are boney outgrowths (osteomas) in the skeleton, and soft tissue tumors. With them present, we have scarcely any need of the evidential support of affected relatives to make the diagnosis. But again, we must be somewhat cautious; for the solitary proband cannot logically be a person who has not yet developed those growths that are outside the colon (which often appear comparatively late). Thus, the probability of being a convincing proband will not be the same for all persons, but will depend on age; and this fact, too, must be kept in mind.

These pitfalls of the proband method tend to make some investigators mistrustful; as a result, they will not try to make any inferences of a probabilistic nature except from standard sampling methods applied to whole populations. However, this policy makes it not only expensive but also prohibitively difficult to study rare diseases, which may well explain why they have been little studied by such methods; for the number of patients examined to find one case may be enormous; the motivation of the unselected subjects (who individually are at low risk) is weak; and the investigator is so bored with examining normal subjects that it is difficult to keep acumen alive. The remedy is, not to run away from the problem, but to capitalize on the proband method, to ensure that the procedure is properly applied, and to carry out the analysis correctly. The technical details (which, though somewhat complicated, ought to be well within the scope of anybody who aspires to be a professional collector of data) would be inappropriate here.

Example 3.5. However, let us deal with a classical problem in genetics (19). Consider some very conspicuous, autosomal, recessive trait that is always recognized and diagnosed; it is also so debilitating that those affected have no progeny, and thus the parents of virtually all cases are carriers. Then every sibship at risk will be discovered provided at least one child in it is affected. Each child of such parents is at a risk of ¼ of being affected. In figure 3.2 we see some simple patterns. If there is only one child, then three-

A. One-child family

B. Two-children family

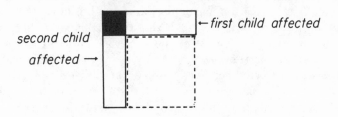

C. Three-children family

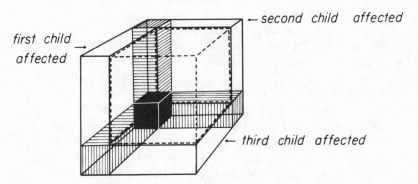

Figure 3.2. Ascertainment bias in the offspring of two parents, both carriers for a recessive Mendelian trait. Each child is at risk of one-fourth of being affected. For a family to be ascertained, at least one child must be affected. The proportion of families *not* ascertained is, in each case, shown by the dashed lines. *A:* There is only one child in the family, who must be affected (*black*), and ¾ of the families are missed. *B:* The first or second child may be affected (*white* rectangles), or both may be (the *black* square at their intersection). Thus, 9/16 of the families are missed. *C:* The first, second, or third child may be affected (the *white* walls and floor), or any two (the *hachured* junctions of the walls), or all three (the *black* cube at the intersection of all three). So 27/64 of families are missed.

quarters of the couples will not be discovered, and of the remaining one-quarter (naturally) all their progeny are affected. If there are two children, the probability of both being unaffected is $(\frac{3}{4})^2$; the first child will be affected, the second unaffected, with probability of $(\frac{1}{4})(\frac{3}{4}) = \frac{3}{16}$; the same probability will apply to the case where the first is unaffected and the second affected; and the probability of both being affected is $(\frac{1}{4})^2 = \frac{1}{16}$. Thus, all told, $\frac{7}{16}$ of the couples will be recognized, and of *their* children, $\frac{4}{7}$ will be affected. If there are three children in the sibship, the couples will not be discovered if all three children are unaffected, which has a probability of $(\frac{3}{4})^3 = \frac{27}{64}$. The couple will be ascertained if any of the three children is affected or any pair or all three, a probability of $\frac{37}{64}$, and the proportion of *their* children affected will be $\frac{16}{37}$. These three proportions, (1), ($\frac{4}{7}$), and ($\frac{16}{37}$), are all related to the basic proportion of $\frac{1}{4}$; but each is differently distorted by the process of ascertainment. What matters is that the nature and impact of the bias is precisely known, and with appropriate adjustments they lead to reliable estimates of the true segregation ratio.

The Reference Population

In a sense, we may regard the foregoing example as illustrating the importance of defining the population of reference and what its properties are. Too often the sampling procedure may pass muster, but it is not at all clear what the population of reference may be. The problem may be simply vagueness, a romantic belief that a haphazard collection of bits and pieces constitutes a random sample. I have deplored this error in chapter 1, and I shall not labor the point. Defining the reference set is of cardinal importance. But one often encounters perfectly well-defined groups in which the notion of a population is elusive, and even effectively meaningless.

Example 3.6. Consider, for instance, the students admitted to medical school. A number of features are clear. There is no claim that the mechanism by which they are selected is a random process. The school will select what it deems the most accomplished students that apply. It may be argued that (in some sense) selection of the candidates that apply to a school and constitute the reference set is random. But then the selection is not a random process applied to a fixed population, but a deliberative process applied to a random population. But there are other oddities. For most selection committees apply neither independent selection nor a uniform set of criteria, but deliberately try to cultivate heterogeneity with the hope that the diverse accomplishments and talents of the students will be mutually enriching. In the light of this pattern, it is difficult to imagine what the class attained by such a selection is supposed to be representative of. However, there is no reason why the group, once selected, should not be regarded as a population about which statements could be made or from which samples might be selected. Whether any conclusion to which such studies might lead has any general (and therefore scientific) value is a complicated matter that I have tried to grapple with elsewhere (12).

CONFOUNDING

The Latin verb *confundere* means "to pour together." We are familiar with the words *fusion* (as in cells or nuclei) and *confusion* (as in politics). Related to them, and especially to the latter, is the word *confound,** which in the eighteenth century was a term of invective, but which in science has assumed a metaphorical and nonabusive meaning. It is applied to the effects of two or more manipulations administered in such a way that no explicit conclusion can be reached about either separately. No great harm is done if one keeps to conclusions about this *combined* effect. But the unwary may fall into inferential traps.

Note a nicety of both grammar and logic. If we have two simultaneous manipulations, A and B, so that their effects exhibit confounding, there is a perfect logical *symmetry* between them; and to represent this grammatically we say their effects are confounded. To call A a "confounding variable" (even if our interest lies only in B) destroys the sense of this reciprocity and has been known to lead to unsound inferences. Moreover, it is not the *variables* that are confounded, but their *effects.*

Example 3.7. Thorn (20) has given a good example of what seems to be confounding. In the early days of the treatment of Addison's disease (a disorder in which the adrenal glands are more or less destroyed), it was thought that epinephrine (a product of the medulla of the gland) might be the lifesaving principle. The drug was administered by enema, and it was considered wisest to give it in dilute form. To avoid osmotic effects, it was given dissolved in normal saline. From this treatment there was indeed an improvement in the patient; but subsequent, more refined studies proved that the epinephrine has little lasting effect. Thorn concludes that

---

*This perception and treatment of *confounding* is logical, and is related only by analogy to the formalized use of the term in orthodox statistics.

it was the saline in which it was given that produced the benefit. Modern understanding of the disorder is that it is the destruction of the *cortex* of the glands that is the main cause of the symptoms, mediated in large part through depletion of sodium throughout the body. Here then, the effects of epinephrine and those of sodium chloride and the other electrolytes in the solvent were confounded. The correct fashion in which to have explored the effect of the treatment would have been to do control studies with the saline solvent alone.

It is not always so easy to separate the effects. The safeguard is then to keep a perpetually suspicious mind as to what a putative treatment is mixed up with. For instance, one may be unable to separate the main effect from an interaction.

Example 3.8. To study effects of dietary cholesterol requires that it be dissolved in special solvent (usually fat), because it cannot be dissolved in water. One may try treatment with the solvent alone. But the difference between the effects of solvent alone and (solvent + cholesterol) may not soundly be ascribed to cholesterol alone: it may be that the solvent itself plays some vital part other than acting as a solvent. For instance, two chemicals equally good as solvents might give very different effects.

One could quote other, far more embarrassing, cases in which one can show from first principles that it is impossible to design an experiment that will resolve such confounding (11). It is not my aim in this book to deal with the experimenter's problems in this or any other such cases, or with how to decide whether or not they can be resolved. But readers will do well to keep constantly probing for weaknesses in an argument. One should not be overwhelmed by what are merely minor flaws in reasoning. The soundness of the conclusion may be in little doubt, despite technical quibbles. However, there is no room for complacency; and the critical reader will draw his own conclusions if a loophole in the evidence has been expressly pointed out but the challenge to remedy it is ignored.

Example 3.9. A familiar illustration is the confounding of the action of a drug with the effect of suggestion, or with some special care that the treated subjects, but not the control subjects, receive. It may also be confounded with the unconscious biases of the observer who (for one reason or another) expects, or hopes for, some effect from the treatment. It is the former problem that has led to the use of the placebo: the patients are *blinded* (kept in ignorance of whether they are receiving the treatment or the placebo). The problem of observer bias is dealt with by blinding the observer as well. It will be obvious that such double-blind experiments cannot be maintained if the treatment has side effects that cannot be masked or simulated in the control group.

Methods of Dealing with Confounding

Confounding can sometimes be kept under control by simple design. But when it is not so easily handled, or where one is unable to conduct experiments and must be content with passive observations (e.g., vital statistics), there are a number of methods of analysis that may be used.

Example 3.10. It is a common experience that certain genetic disorders are more likely in children born to elderly parents. Now, broadly, the two spouses tend to be of similar ages. So if we observe the child born to elderly, but healthy, parents, what was the important factor? Was it the mother's age? The father's? Or did it operate only if both were elderly? Was it the year of birth of one parent or the other? Was it related to the social prosperity of the parents? Was there an ascertainment bias? (For instance, older parents usually have more experience of caring for children than younger parents do, and they would more readily identify abnormality of behavior or of development.)

The methods of adjustment for confounding—mainly multiple covariance analysis and stratification—are well known among statisticians. They make it possible to do the equivalent of holding one possible factor constant so that the effect of the other may be inferred. Covariance analysis is too technical to discuss here. But the reader should know that it exists and that it is the business of the conscientious investigator to use it when appropriate.

Stratification. It might seem that experiments are best done on homogeneous classes (e.g., inbred mice). Gratuitous variation would be small; tests powerful; conclusions clean. But there are two snags. Strictly speaking, any conclusions would not apply to other species or even to all mice. Second, human groups would rarely be suitable for such experiments. A common compromise is to reduce variation within groups by grouping subjects into strata. The subsequent analysis, though more complex and not discussed here, may be helpful. Readers will have two concerns, however.

First, How are the strata formed. They may be natural, e.g., genotype or sex. They may be arbitrary, e.g., grouping by ages 30–34, 35–39, etc. Variation within the stratum must be presumed to be small. The narrower the strata, the more sound this belief; but also the fewer patients will fall into each stratum.

The harder problem is to express the result. At times the breach due to stratification cannot be healed. The hormone LSH raises the blood progesterone level in women; but not in men, who do not ovulate. No statement, unqualified by sex, can be made about how all adults respond to LSH. By contrast, at all ages, in all races, and for both sexes, increasing the proportion of saturated fat in the diet raises the serum cholesterol level; so a simple, broad statement is sound. But often there is increase in some strata and decrease in others, partly from sampling error, partly from true differences. Formalistic statisticians may tidy such results up by invoking "interactions." Serum cholesterol seems to rise with age, but it crests earlier in men; and statisticians would say that age and sex interact. But biologists should not think that such a mathematical interaction between them implies a biochemical one. A neat formula for the expected combined effect of age and sex may be convenient in the clinic. But the symbols in it may have no biological counterpart. Indeed, statisticians may also use mathematical devices for removing statistical interactions, but in so doing, they clearly are not changing the biochemistry of the body! While one can form a hazy idea of a simple interaction, it gets steadily harder to imagine a higher-order interaction (e.g., among age, sex, race, and occupation) or to see how it suggests the next line of enquiry.

My aim in this brief note is not to turn readers against stratification but to point out that it may lead to misunderstanding, and that finding the meaning (as distant from its descriptive utility) is best left to mathematically sophisticated biologists.

AMBIGUITY

Finally, we must address a problem of science which is rarely confronted explicitly, but which is becoming progressively more disruptive. The three great tools of communication are diagrams, symbols, and language. In certain circles it is fashionable to say that they are all much the same thing; but it is rare to find anybody even modestly accomplished in the use of all three, and I am led to believe that they are more or less separate. Mathematical symbols (e.g., birth weight) are quite different from poetic symbols,* not so much in how true they are as in how they are true. Medicine has its share of poetry—in origin, a muscle is *a little mouse,* a tissue *something that has been spun;* a person is an actor's mask through which the inner being *sounds.*

The mathematical aspect of Medicine waxes and wanes: at

---

*A beloved would look ludicrous if her lips were indeed rubies and her cheeks roses—thorns and all.

present it is vigorous in the field of measurement, but rather neglected as a method of formal reasoning. Diagrams are in wide use to express simple relationships; but anything adventurous tends to repel the fainthearted. Carelessly used, all three tools are apt to lead to ambiguity, which is only rarely deliberate; and the ambiguity is at times perilous.

Words

I shall not discuss English grammar or the vital art of consulting dictionaries; but I do protest at the horrors that come from their neglect. The "bold, plain, style" is to be commended. The main defense for technical vocabulary is that, properly used, *it prevents ambiguity.* This end is impeded by malapropisms. (I wonder how often most readers consult a dictionary? But it is a wasted refinement unless the writers too are faithful to the dictionary.)

Invented words do little to help.

Example 3.11. Having puzzled in a paper over the abbreviation *u.i.d.,* I concluded that it meant "once a day." But the Latin word for once (if one must use Latin) is *semel;* and even to use the abbreviation *s.i.d.* is perilous. If brevity is the issue, *daily* uses five symbols against six in the abbreviation.

There are less happy outcomes. I have seen on a diabetic's chart of urine tests the abbreviation *ns,* which I took to mean "no sugar" whereas it meant "no specimen," an ambiguity that nearly brought me to grief. I would point out that there is nothing more parochial than abbreviations. In London *p.i.d.* commonly means "prolapsed intervertebral disc," whereas in Baltimore it means "pelvic inflammatory disease," a serious source of misunderstanding, especially in a patient with backache.

There is a more diffuse ambiguity that comes from a kind of general woolliness of style. One fault is an overuse of abstract words and clumsy prefabricated phrases. According to this cant, patients (or cases?) are not operated on, they "have surgery." An urgent need is called "an emergency situation." A second fault is the use of vague demonstratives when their antecedents are unclear. I have come to avoid altogether the use of *this* and *that* as pronouns. A third is a careless use of metaphor. Many sentences are ambiguous for stylistic reasons. Are "vital data" those got during life? Or are they essential to establish a conclusion? Or are they derived from national statistics? (If readers think that I am creating difficulties out of nothing, I assure them that on one occasion I have had a paper rejected for publication because a reviewer supposed that by the word *vital* I meant "logically important," whereas I meant it in its literal sense, "living" as distinct from "chemical." The misunderstanding was successfully resolved.)

Conceptual Ambiguity

It would be a false emphasis to suppose that all ambiguity is verbal and may be avoided by attention to grammar and style. More important (because more insidious) is ambiguity of ideas. Many people have hazy recollections from Dryden and Pope that genius and madness are "near allied." They mistake the confusion of the two states by mediocre minds for a true relationship between them, as if madness were an occupational disease among scholars. One might as well suppose that because bronchial spasm (bronchial asthma) and paroxysmal left ventricular failure (cardiac asthma) are often confused, there must be some nontrivial causal relationship between them.

An overhasty choice of the key feature of a problem or the use of a lay term to designate it are two particularly dangerous sources of ambiguity.

Example 3.12. Take the word *fitness.* In the lay mind it calls up a vision of athletes and middle-aged joggers. Yet this image has nothing to do with whether someone is fit to be in charge of a university. A squalid fame overtook the word when the pamphleteers (like Robert W. Service and the lesser Darwinians) took to using *Fitness* as a mystical term akin to *Progress.* Biological *fitness* was rescued from total semantic emptiness by population geneticists when they used it to denote the "average size of completed family." And others have used it to mean the probability that a particular genetic line will not become extinct. Now while they are usually somewhat related, there is no clear correspondence between any pair of these meanings (21); and none of them has any heuristic meaning at all. The only fact assured by a large average size of family is that on average the size of the family will be large. This fact tells us something (but not everything) about whether the family is likely to die out; but it tells nothing at all about its fitness in other senses; about whether it will consist of athletes or weaklings, whether they will be worthy of public office, whether their clothes will be the right size, or whether they are epileptics. As Li (22) penetratingly pointed out, eugenic statements such as that the unfit may propagate widely and flood the gene pool show a hopeless confusion of terms. This whole intellectual quagmire is traceable to the superficial and empty slogan about "the survival of the fittest"; the increasingly desperate efforts to give it some meaning; and the unhappy endowment of a common word with a lofty meaning. And not even a sound lay term: men may run faster miles, but women live longer.

Evidential Ambiguity

The ambiguity may lie, not in faulty expression or in confused invention, but in the sources of evidence that we seek to interpret. I mean by this distinction that interpreting what somebody intends to convey (*communicative meaning*) is not necessarily, perhaps not at all, the same as discovering what is to be inferred from what we perceive in nature (*illative meaning*). Puzzling out what somebody means by saying "Put that in the other one in there" (23) is not the same as trying to discover why the dinosaur died out. Analysis will readily persuade us that "boys will be boys," "the advances due to progress," and "the rarity of exceptional people" are phrases that have no thought content; but at least the speaker who used these phrases believed that they did and yearned to share his imitation thoughts with us. We are not sure that, in the same sense, a spinning top is trying to tell us something.

We may learn something about physiology from solving an equation; but an equation may have multiple solutions (or "roots"), some of which we may be able to discard as meaningless. For instance, we cannot have a gene frequency of 150 percent, a negative mortality rate, or an imaginary cardiac output. However, there may be multiple roots that are all intelligible, and the data we have may be insufficient to provide a unique answer.

By analogy, much of the clinical endeavor is shrouded in ambiguity. A relationship between two quantities, X and Y, is said to be monotonic if an increase in X is always accompanied by a rise, or is accompanied by a fall, in Y; and conversely for decrease. Thus, the relationship between the height of a man and the length of the shadow he casts (even on rough ground) is monotonic (fig. 3.3). But many biological patterns are not of this form.

Example 3.13. The cardiac output may decrease when the venous pressure is either too low (as in shŏck) or too high (as in heart failure).

Example 3.14. Nephritis may lead to either a very high output of urine, or to no output at all.

The diagnostician may find it difficult to distinguish the prime disorder from a response of the body to the exactly opposite state.

Example 3.15. A cold sweat may be associated with a *high* blood sugar level in pheochromocytoma (a tumor that causes a purposeless output of nonadrenaline); a cold sweat may also be associ-

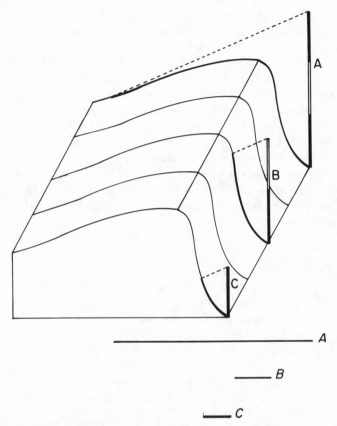

Figure 3.3. A monotonic relationship. The heights of the three poles, *A*, *B*, and *C*, are in the proportions 3:2:1. The top of each is connected by a dashed line to the tip of its shadow. The ground is not level, but has the same cross section at all positions along its axis. The lengths of the shadows are shown by the lines below. They are not proportional to the heights of the poles, but the tallest pole has the longest shadow, and conversely, the shortest the shortest. For lengths in between, one could not at once say what the correct heights of the poles are, but one could arrange them in correct order. (Reproduced from Edmond A. Murphy, "Only authorized persons admitted: The quantitative genetics of health and disease," *John Hopkins Medical Journal* 148:114–22, 1981, by kind permission of the editor.)

ated with a *low* blood sugar (e.g., due to an overdose of insulin), which the adrenal gland is stimulated to combat.

As to prognosis, a fairly low white cell count in blood during a fever may be a reassuring sign (the infection is well under control) or a sinister one (the patient can respond no better). Likewise, loss of a fever in cholera may mean that the patient is recovering; or entering the "algid" (i.e., shocked) stage. In therapeutics, the patient given digoxin may be nauseated because the dosage is inadequate or because it is excessive (although for quite different reasons in the two cases). During general anesthesia with ether, the pupils may be enlarged and the breathing arrested either because the level of anesthesia is too light or too deep.

I do not say that these ambiguities defy solution (in the same way as the ambiguity of the equation does); but they exist and may call for the greatest perceptiveness on the part of the clinician. The danger lies in failing to realize that many relationships in biology do not have a clear and simple trend throughout. Because one dosage is good for you, a dosage ten times as large is not necessarily ten times better for you, a lesson that is obvious—but often, and painfully, forgotten.

PROBLEMS

3.1. Confirm the conclusions reached for figure 3.2.
3.2. Criticize the following sentences.
    a. The last thing a nervous patient should do is make a will.
    b. Achondroplasts should be persuaded to have smaller families.
    c. Neglect of infected teeth may lead to defective nutrition. This may be reflected in indigestion and a blotchy complexion, calling for expert intervention which is most undesirable.
    d. In SBE persistent fever may be the tip of the iceberg; specific treatment calls for broad-spectrum antibiotics given parentally. If nauseous, the nursing staff should inform the physician.
3.3. Dogs hunt lizards; lizards catch insects; insects spread infectious disease among dogs. What would be the effect on dogs of a massive destruction of insects?
3.4. Consider the impact of publications dealing with the phenotype of the XYY karyotype on the obstacles to further elucidation of the phenotypic effects of this karyotype.
3.5. A survey on the frequency of schizophrenia is conducted by confidential questionnaire sent through the mails to be filled in by the individual person. The following groups are studied:
    a. A random sample of the population
    b. The alumni of a liberal arts college who graduated between 1935 and 1940

    c.   Board-certified American psychiatrists

    d.   United States Congressmen

    e.   Geneticists.

    Consider how you would interpret the results.

3.6. The extremes of bias come from those who have insight into their bigotries and call them principles. Comments?

3.7. The importance of education to society is largely championed by the writings of the educated. The illiterate do not write books on the unimportance of education. Does this argument mean that collective views about education are biased? If so, is that a reason for discounting them?

3.8. Cows have now been bred that have such a high yield of milk as to make them deficient in calcium. Calcium-deficiency is, of course, harmful, even fatal. By the Darwinian criterion of survival of a genetic line, does this genetic pattern make these animals more fit or less? (Careful!)

Part **II** Probability and
Statistics

4 | Variation

Science exists because things vary with some regularity. Thus, whatever their scientific background, clinicians can be no strangers to variation. We shall discuss the nature of variation in greater detail in chapter 7. Here we shall be content with a somewhat formalistic treatment.

In science it is necessary to think in terms of two kinds of variation.

Mathematical Variation

We mean by this term the variation in magnitude of the attributes of the stable structures of experience. The atomic weights of elements vary, for instance. Species vary in the number of chromosomes per cell they ordinarily have. Metals vary in their specific gravities. The quantities involved are all definite enough to merit compilation in handbooks and other reference sources. There is no component of caprice in these values. We do not for a moment imagine that on Mars the atomic weight of oxygen is forty or that in some foreign country the human beings usually have fifty-six chromosomes.

Random Variation

Yet we also encounter variation that in the individual datum cannot be predicted with perfect precision. This random variation is mostly of three common forms.

1. Experimental error. Try as one may, the hand shakes, the eyes blur, one mistimes an event. This kind of variation is merely a source of embarrassment to the scientist, and he tries to keep it as small as possible.

2. Those who go on to study nuclear physics or biology soon realize that however much refinement is introduced into experiments, there is a practical, perhaps inescapable and intrinsic, limit to the predictability of the outcome. In the use of radionuclides this variation is familiar. The variation in blood pressure or blood cholesterol from day to day, even under the most carefully standardized conditions that can be devised, is far greater than that due to error of measurement. Some of the variation may be circadian (i.e., repeating a systematic pattern every twenty-four hours) or seasonal; but not all of it is; and while there are those who believe that with a sufficiently detailed analysis of factors one could account for all the variation, nobody has in fact succeeded in doing so. It remains an act of faith that it can be done, even in principle. This residual variation is mostly regarded as an inescapable nuisance.

3. But a third kind of random variation is not a nuisance but positive evidence of some effect of interest. This type is well exemplified in genetics.

Example 4.1. If the degree of variation in a trait is greater between "unlike" than "like" twins, we may tentatively infer that there are genetic factors contributing to the treatment.

Example 4.2. The Lyon hypothesis (24)—that in each body cell all but one X chromosome becomes inactive—is triumphantly supported by the fact that the amount and pattern of the random variation predicted by it is in fact observed.

Thus, the authentic biologist who begins with the idea that statements of measurement should be exact to six significant figures comes to tolerate, and eventually to welcome, random variation.

THE NATURE OF RANDOM VARIATION

But we are going a little too fast. The perceptive reader may feel that I have glossed over the ambiguities in my terms. Systematic effects are easy enough to accept because we are, or think we are, accustomed to seeing them. But a random effect: Is this merely an evasive term we use to hide pure ignorance? Or are we trying to invest randomness with an identity that is outside our ordinary notion of scientific causality? Or is it something that nobody really believes in, but is a convenient fiction, like John Doe or the Reasonable Man? Is it merely an unsightly intellectual scaffolding that we use for the time being while we are grappling with the major factors, and which later on we intend to remove? I wish it were possible to state a consensus; but in fact most people seem to be shy about expressing any exact opinion on the point. Many of the probabilists seem to be content to make the purely formal statement that a random effect is one that has a probability distribution, and to express no opinion at all as to what that may mean in scientific terms, or in mechanisms of production. Some physical theorists seem to regard the characteristics of randomness as an ultimate physical reality: an electron *is* a probability distribution. Some biologists believe that, in principle, every last detail can be accounted for, even the components of experimental error. Some applied statisticians seem to think of randomness as like an iceberg melting in the warm sea of scientific enquiry: it will eventually all disappear, but in the meantime the scientist is buoyed up by it. The latter viewpoint seems to involve using proofs, which all would agree are probabilistic, to demolish probability as a notion; I confess that I am very uncomfortable over the soundness and consistency of that idea. It seems to argue that having climbed up on a proof, one can, as it were, kick the proof out from underfoot without losing one's poise.

My own scientific opinion, for what it is worth, is that there probably is an escapable minimum indeterminacy in the physical world that cannot be reduced to causal mechanisms. However, unlike chaos (with which it is often confused, even sometimes by the sophisticated), this randomness has a corporate regularity that can be described.

Example 4.3. The movements of individual gas molecules may be random, but the collective behavior of a container full of them will obey standard gas laws (as every anesthetist or specialist in pulmonary diseases knows).

Much that is at present ascribed to randomness will eventually prove to be predictable as knowledge increases. But we should beware of the naive assumption that the effective magnitude of random effects is no greater than that of subatomic particles. (The latter effects, because of mutual independence, tend in large part to cancel each other out.) As I have remarked elsewhere, the predictability of the direction of a stampede of cattle is by no means so clear as we would expect if each animal behaved independently (12). The kinetic theory of gases does not apply to the behavior of a crowd in a fire. The indeterminacy in the human behavior that we call free will, and which used to seem to be such a thorn in the flesh of the physicist, may have an analogous origin.

Example 4.4. Macfarlane's famous cascade theory of coagulation (25) showed how a small initial random effect may be amplified by the intermediate steps of the process and lead to a massive end response.

I hope that the reader will form a mature personal theory of randomness and not suppose that anything either in theory or in practice compels allegiance to any doctrinaire opinions.

ON CHARACTERIZING VARIATION

The Empiricist's Perspective

If it be granted that at least some variation is an authentic but unpredictable feature of particular events and processes, how can we describe it? The most natural and the safest way is to observe what happens in a large number (say 10,000) of independent* instances, sort them out into arbitrary classes, and find out how many observations fall within each class. Such a display (fig. 4.1) is called a *histogram*. However, we are in some difficulty here; for the notion that a random process can be described, and that it exhibits regularity, means that if we collect another set of data and handle it in the same way, the histograms should have the same shape; but this belief would not square completely with the idea of random independent behavior of each individual reading. If at some stage in collecting the second sample the quota in an individual class (as set by the first sample) is filled, then if the exact same shapes in the two histograms are to result, all future sample values must belong to other classes. This restriction of choices is progressive; and eventually there would be no options left for the ten-thousandth value in the second histogram. This last event would not be random, or the histograms would not be certainly identical. Either way, we end with a contradiction.

We are led to the conclusion that the randomness in the observations implies randomness in the form of the histogram. What then has become of our claim that the randomness exhibits regularity? This: that (suitably scaled) the undoubted variability of the entire histogram is much less than the variability of the individual observations; and that (suitably scaled) the larger the sample of observations, the smaller the variability. Eventually the histogram settles down to a fixed pattern that is the description we are seeking. The random quantity we are studying is the *random variable* or *variate*. The idealized histogram approached by an ever larger sample grouped into ever narrower classes is its *probability distribution*.

---

*In probability algebra, *independence* has a technical meaning. *A* and *B* are independent if the probability that they both happen is the product of the probabilities of their happening individually. This claim cannot be verified empirically for any *individual* pair of events. In practice, meeting this assumption is largely a matter of common sense.

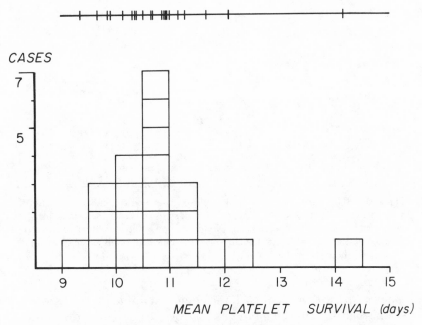

Figure 4.1. On a line (*top*) are marked off the individual estimates of the mean survival of blood platelets in twenty-one subjects with untreated gout (data of Smythe et al., 3). They are represented in the *lower* diagram, grouped by intervals of half a day to form a histogram. Each appears in the histogram as an individual square. (In practice, it is not usual to mark off individual cases by the horizontal lines in each column, which are shown here merely in the interests of clarity.)

The Probabilist's Perspective

Now a modern probabilist would have a somewhat different way of looking at a probability distribution. The reader may not find this second, mathematical, conception to be of much help to him personally; but for purposes of communication, if for no other reason, it is well to be aware of the argument. The probabilist argues that for one thing, one never can obtain infinite samples, so that the approach through the histogram is not practicable. Second, if each sample value is denoted by a unit area, the bigger the sample, the bigger the histogram; but the probability distribution (which is a statement about a population) cannot grow with the size of the sample any more than the size of the moon would depend on the number of observations we made of it; by convention, the probability of an event cannot exceed unity (that is, certainty), and it would be necessary to rescale the histogram according to the size of the sample. Third, a histogram always consists of a set of rec-

ANASCOPESIS   PROGNOSIS   PROJECTION

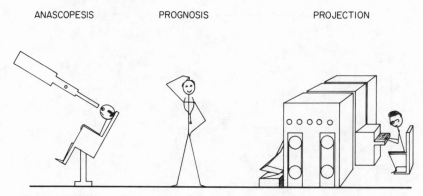

Figure 4.2. Three activities of medical scientists. Anascopesis (hindsight) consists of analyzing experience; it is the central concern of statistics. Prognosis (foresight), the main goal of probability algebra, deals with prediction in the individual case. Projection (a major activity of biomathematics) is a more or less sophisticated integration of fact and theory to make sound generalizations.

tangles, and the width of each rectangle will influence the shape of the histogram. But the mind gibes at the idea of letting the nature of the probabilities depend on so irrelevant an issue as *how we have arbitrarily chosen to group the data.*

Probabilists deal with these problems by taking a different stance. They see a distribution as a predictive statement about the respective plausibilities of the various *possible* outcomes from any *single future* execution of the random process. In forming such a statement, they will appeal both to empirical science and to general theoretical knowledge. But to them, a distribution is not merely a compilation of experiences, which a histogram is. The probabilist is, as it were, looking forward (prognosis), as the clinician is; the statistician is looking backwards (anascopesis), as the student of populations is (fig. 4.2). There is nothing very revolutionary about this probabilistic view of a process; nevertheless, it may be temporarily upsetting when first encountered. Perhaps a familiar example will help.

Example 4.5. Suppose that a woman is known to be a carrier of hemophilia. What is the probability that her next son will be affected? The answer is ½. How are we to see this answer?

Clearly it is not a statement about a proportion in this woman's next 10,000 sons. She will have only a few sons altogether; in fact she will have only one *next* son. So, large-sample interpretations are useless. Furthermore, the statement cannot be based on experience even of her one next son, because he does not yet exist. (If he did,

there would be no point in merely predicting whether he is affected when, to be certain, we merely have to examine him.) Then
how do we know that the answer is ½? And what does the answer
mean?

As to the first question, we appeal (rightly or wrongly) to two
sources. First, a Mendelian theory of the carrier state of an X-
linked trait, the paired nature of chromosomes, and the equal
probabilities that the two members of the mother's pair of X chromosomes will be inherited. Second, extensive experience that the
proportion of hemophilic sons born to carrier mothers does indeed
conform to the Mendelian pattern. In other words, it is a mixture
of reasonable argument and sound corroborative data about *a class
of similar problems*.

What the answer means is a more elusive matter. In a practical
situation such as genetic counseling, one commonly lends perspective to the risk by comparing it with the risk unselected mothers
(whether knowingly or not) take in any pregnancy. In unselected
pregnancies, about one child in forty is born with a serious physical
abnormality. The fact that this woman is a carrier of hemophilia
means that the risk is increased about tenfold. That is, one may
think of probabilities in terms of individual gambles. An insurance
broker would not (like the mother) think in individual pregnancies
but in terms of to what proportion of a particular class of pregnancies the insurance company may expect to pay out; that is, he is
thinking in terms of what we called the empiricist's perspective.
The probabilist would argue that a probability is an abstract intuitive notion that does not need to be interpreted, any more than
equality or identity do. I leave it to readers to make their own
interpretations.

However, I think it helps to see the theory and the practical
reality, *not as attempts to describe the same thing, but as an exercise in
congruity*. It is like the relationship between footwear and the man-
ufacturing of shoes. In mass production one does not set out to
make an individual shoe for each foot. Nor, on the other hand, do
we try to cram a foot into a stereotyped shoe. Rather what happens
is that the manufacturer has to develop a theory about the class of
feet to be accommodated. It has to meet four classes of constraints.
First, it must have some structural coherence; there are limits on
how a sound shoe may be built; and these demands are like the
axioms of the probabilist. Second, it must be apt: an elegant theory
may lead to shoes that fit nobody. Third, it is influenced by what we
may call pentheric demands: the theory must have a certain simplicity, economy, plausibility. The shoe must be agreeable to look

at. It must be easy to keep clean and polish. Fourth, it must have a normative character. One of the functions of shoes, for instance, is to correct fallen arches: the shoemaker does not merely make a shoe that will fit snugly even if the result is highly pathological. On the other hand, he is not trying by hook or by crook to force the foot to conform to some highly arbitrary ideal.

The notion that should emerge from this analogy is that the theory is not merely casting in bronze what the empirical data cast in clay, or conversely. The theoretical and the empirical are two different entities with different contents, different allegiances, different standards, different contributions toward our understanding. But if they are both competently pursued, they will lead to a certain degree of congruity, and the discrepancies should lead both to further enquiries that will promote further harmonies. Broadly, theory furnishes shape; practice lends authenticity. It is an abuse to treat theory as a little fancy decoration added at the last moment to make a crassly empirical study suitable to be published in The Best Journals. Nor should a theory so crush an experiment that the scientists' perception is distorted. The readers (my audience) more than anybody should cultivate a sense of this harmony. To extend the metaphor, the statistician gives much thought to how far his model will stretch without doing violence to the data to which it is applied. A model that will stretch is said to be *robust*.

We have cause to be concerned at those who confuse these roles. In discussing how something should behave in actuality, they say on the one hand that "Theory shows that. . . ." The odds are that theory does not. It is almost never in a position to do so. In view of its allegiances, all the strict conclusions to which theory leads lie within the domain of pure theory. Of its kind, a theory may be excellent, but it may have nothing to do with the real world. If theory proves something contrary to the facts, so much the worse for the theory. On the other hand, the dyed-in-the-wool empiricist has a habit of appealing to a body of data and adding "I am only trying to be logical." That is one thing that he is not doing. Empirical, yes. Reasonable, perhaps. But logic is an abstract relationship among agreed principles. It has nothing whatsoever to do with whether something is true or not. As Whitehead pointed out (26), the big flaw in medieval science was that it supposed that reasoning is an adequate substitute for observation. A big temptation in modern biology is the exact opposite: to suppose that more and more facts measured to more and more decimal places will circumvent the need for coherent theory and logical argument. One of the perils of abandoning all theory is precisely that it leaves one impervious to the demonstrated failures of the past. One confuses truth with validity and reasoning with empirical fact.

REPRESENTATION OF A DISTRIBUTION

A distribution may be represented in a variety of abstract mathematical ways. But many scientists (myself included) find it much easier to think in terms of images. Earlier in this chapter, we have pictured probability as proportional to area in a diagram; but in a distribution we have to think of a scale of value as well. Any pictorial representation is a set of conventions. So I shall stick to the convention that *area represents probability*.

Figure 4.3A pictures a conventional target with three concentric circles. The bull's eye has an area of one unit; the inner, an area of three; and the outer, an area of five. The total target has an area of nine units, the outer framework, representing the sample space, has an area of thirty units. Suppose that an arrow is shot absolutely blind, so that *all directions are equally likely*. Granted that the arrow falls within the frame, there is a probability of 9/30 that the target will be hit; of 3/30 = 1/10 that the inner will be hit; and so on.

We may make *conditional* probability statements. *If* the target (nine units) is hit, *then* the probability that the bull's eye is also hit is 1/9.

If there are two targets (fig. 4.3B), the smaller having a total area of four units and a bull's eye of two units, we can make comparisons between the probabilities of competing explanations. If we know that one target or the other has been hit but we do not know which, the odds are nine to four that it was the left-hand one that was hit. If one bull's eye was hit, the odds are two to one that it was the one on the right. This latter kind of comparison illustrates *Bayes' theorem*. It takes into consideration the relative sizes of the targets (*prior probabilities*) and the relative proportions of the two targets taken up by their bull's eyes (*conditional probabilities*).

Discrete Variables

Example 4.6. Consider the rather odd-looking target in figure 4.4A. Again, an arrow is shot at it in such a way that all points on the target are equally likely to be hit, and complete misses are ignored. To hit the square counts 1; the rectangle, 2; the parallelogram, 3; and the lozenge, 4. Hits elsewhere count as 0. The probability of a particular outcome will be proportional to area. Thus, to represent the corresponding distribution, we might simply cut out these figures and arrange them on a scale; but since one

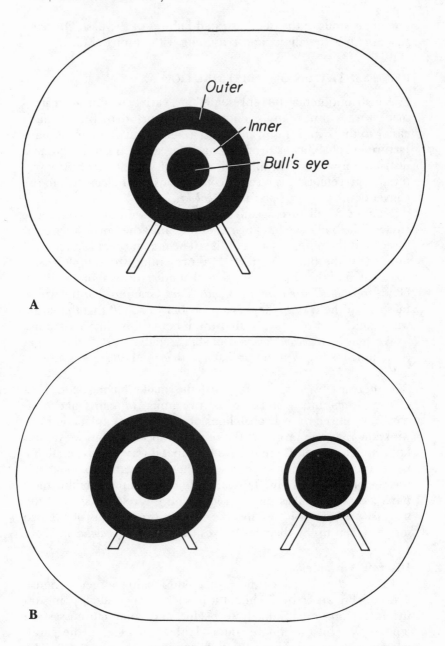

Figure 4.3. Probability algebra as targetry. *A:* A target seen as an event in a sample space. The bull's eye is ⅟₃₀ of the total space. *B:* A second, nonoverlapping target is added to the same sample space. Its bull's eye is twice as large, but its total area is the same as the inner two areas of the first target.

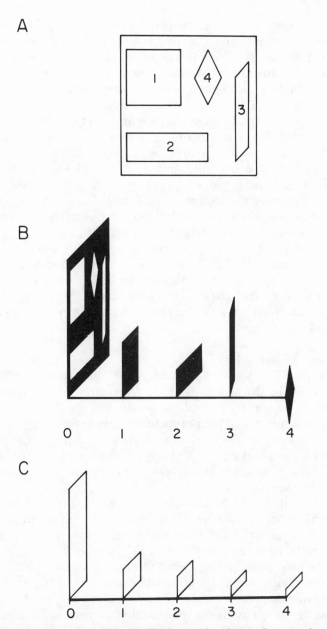

Figure 4.4. A discrete probability distribution. Each point on the target is equally likely to be hit, so that area is proportional to probability. *A:* The sectors of various shapes have been assigned the scores shown. *B:* The probability distribution. *C:* The distribution has been recast with probabilities shown as rectangles of the same areas as in *B,* but with bases of a constant length. Hence the height is proportional to the probability.

cannot represent an area at a point, in figure 4.4B the areas are displayed at right angles to the axis of measurement ("square-rigged"). Because of the odd shapes, it is not easy to compare the probabilities directly. Therefore *preserving exact areas carefully,* we recast each as a rectangle having the same length of baseline or *footing* (fig. 4.4C). Hence, for each rectangle, the *height,* having no area, is not a probability; but it is proportional to the area, and thus to the probability. The sum of all the areas must obviously add up to one, because when the target is hit, *some* one of the outcomes must occur. Hence, if we add the heights and multiply them by the length of the footing, the result must be unity. We can make it even simpler by giving the footing a unit length. Then we must ensure that the sums of the heights is also unity (the usual check in practice that a discrete distribution is properly scaled).

In example 4.6 there is a definite probability associated with each of the values 0, 1, 2, 3, and 4; but there is no probability for an intermediate value. Such a distribution is said to be *discrete.* For instance, any variate that can be counted is discrete: the number of children in a family (fig. 4.5A); the number of operations a patient has had.

Continuous Variables

Example 4.7. Suppose the variable were "distance in cm from the dead center of the target." The area associated with the value 30 cm would be the area of all the points exactly 30 cm from the center; it is the area of the perimeter of a circle that has a radius of 30 cm. Now the area of a line is zero. Hence, the probability associated with this point is zero! But this result does not mean that the logic of our system has broken down. Let us take the argument a little more slowly.

Suppose that the diameter of the target in figure 4.3A is 60 cm. The probability that the arrow hits between 20 and 40 cm from the center is the area of a band that we have called an inner. We might make the score discrete and say that all inners count as thirty points and produce a probability distribution of the same type as that shown in figure 4.4C. But we could convert the discrete type of scoring into one that scores exactly by distance. To do so, we rotate each of the panels in the discrete distribution so that it is spread out over an interval. By this maneuver we have not abandoned our convention that area means probability; the total area is still unity. We can calculate the probability of a hit between any two distances from the center by finding the area under the curves between these two points. As we noted before, the vertical axis in all these dia-

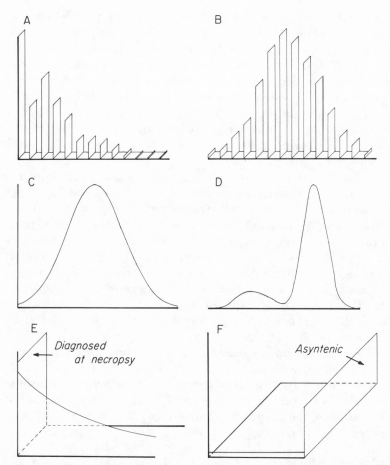

Figure 4.5. Types of distribution. *A:* The number of progeny born to parents with hereditary polyposis coli (27). *B:* Height of British adults, grouped to the nearest inch (28). *C:* The theoretical Gaussian distribution, which is continuous. (The tails, which extend infinitely in both directions, have been cut off.) *D:* A continuous, bimodal distribution. *E:* Hypothetical curve of survival from diagnosis in malignant hypertension, a mixed type of distribution. The main part of the distribution represents the graduated prospects for those alive; the part at right angles represents those already dead. *F:* Prior distribution of genetic linkage, a mixed type of distribution (29).

grams is not probability, but for some length of footing it would generate an area and hence a probability. We call it the *probability density*. In figure 4.4 we converted probability density (height) into probability by multiplying by the length of the footing to give the area of a rectangle. But in a continuous distribution, a segment of the density curve is unlikely to give a perfectly rectangular segment.* Should we wish to change the shape of our distribution in any way, since the total probability must remain one, *we must conserve area.* For instance, if, in order to show more detail, we were to double the horizontal scale, we would have to halve the vertical height. Or if we convert height (in inches) into height (in centimeters) by multiplying by 2.54, we must divide the density by this same factor throughout to conserve the area.

• *Whether or not a distribution is continuous has nothing whatsoever to do with whether it is all in one place.*

A distribution in two or more parts with unoccupied segments between may still be continuous if the number of possible values the data may assume cannot be counted. The pattern in figure 4.5D is a common one. If there is a clear gap between the two parts of the population, there is a common but incorrect custom of calling it discontinuous. In any mathematical context, this term is meaningless. In the model there are no half measures. If the panels are *exactly* at right angles to the baseline and, seen from the front, the mass of each has no spread at all, the distribution is discrete. But if they are rotated by even the slightest amount, they occupy frontage and the distribution is continuous.

Most distributions in biology are continuous. Often, however, we artificially make a continuous variable discrete. Height is a continuous variable: measured with sufficient accuracy, it may assume any value within a reasonable interval. But we often record, not "height," but "height to the nearest inch," which is treating it as discrete (fig. 4.5B).

Mixed Variables

If only the above conventions were adopted ("square-rigging" for discrete variable and "fore-and-aft rigging" for continuous), distributions might be much easier to grasp. But there are other states. As an illustration, consider the case where the distribution is partly continuous and partly discrete. I give two instances.

Example 4.8. What is the distribution of survivorship (length of further survival) from diagnosis in (say) malignant hypertension? The cases we meet are of two types.

1. Some proportion (perhaps 10 percent) are diagnosed at necropsy. The future survival (in this world at least) is zero. Thus at 0 ("no further survival"), there is a lump of probability, 0.1.

---

*However, in representing *sample* data from a continuous variable as a histogram, it is the convention to cast the sample proportion that falls into a class as a rectangle, as in figure 4.5B.

2. The distribution in the remainder, diagnosed in life, is clearly continuous, like all natural events in time.

In conventional diagrams we could not easily portray this pattern. But in figure 4.5E we present the mixture by a square-rigged part and a fore-and-aft rigged part.

Example 4.9. This illustration (fig. 4.5F) will be a familiar one to geneticists. So long as two genetic loci are on different chromosomes, in accordance with Mendel's second law, genes at them inherited from the same parent will have a 50 percent chance of parting company ("recombining") when they are being transmitted to the progeny. If the loci are carried on the *same* chromosome, the probability of recombining may assume any value between 0 and 50 percent, depending on how close together they are. If the probability is less than 50 percent, the loci are said to be linked. Now if I propose to pick any pair of loci at random (but have not yet done so), the probability we would give beforehand of their being on different chromosomes and therefore "unlinked" is about 94 percent.* Thus, the probability distribution will be continuous from recombination values of 0 to 50 percent, with a mass of probability of 0.94 at a recombination value of 50 percent (indicated by the arrow in fig. 4.5F).

CHARACTERIZATION OF A DISTRIBUTION

If the ultimate aim is exactness, the distribution itself cannot in general be improved on. But usually the exact true distribution is not known, and the form of the histogram of experiences will be more or less distorted by the random variation due to sampling and the arbitrary grouping of the results, as we have seen.

One way of reducing this distortion may be to call on a more or less serious background theory as to what the form of the curve may be. But it must be a *serious* theory. There is a common, but totally false, belief that all distributions in "normal" people follow the "normal" (i.e., Gaussian) distribution, shown in figure 4.5C. That is nothing but a feeble pun, like supposing that all political liberals are openhanded with their money. There is no reason whatsoever why normal values should follow any particular form.

Often scientists will use a particular distribution, not because they have any theoretical basis for doing so, but because it seems to fit the data, and they are satisfied that they have enough data to test that claim. This course seems to me quite reasonable, and the more

*This figure is partly empirical. Details are beside the point.

the data, the more reasonable the argument. But there is a golden rule of science that one should be cautious about extrapolating beyond one's experience. The fact that a thousand data fit a particular distribution as well as may be expected from a sample of that size is no warrant for laying down the law about what theory "has shown must happen," and thus has defined what may be dismissed as impossible. All sound conclusions with empirical warrants are inescapably fluid. The distribution and the theory derived from it are not introduced to brutalize the data but to help in a compact but *faithful* description of how the data in fact have behaved. Beyond a certain point, one may abandon one description for another. This point would arrive much later if the provisional model has serious theoretical support.

SIMPLE DESCRIPTORS

For those who want them, a brief account of standard elementary statistics is given in the appendix. There the treatment is mildly technical, and it will have little importance or interest to general readers except those who conscientiously propose to check the conclusions in papers they read. What follows is directed to the conception and meaning of some statistical descriptors, and how they relate to the nontechnical inspection made by the intelligent reader when confronted with a set of data.

The scientist is sometimes reluctant to use any particular distribution (because experience is too slight, and he has no adequate theory). Yet the data may still be too unwieldy to think about usefully as individual items. Then the question arises of how the data can be "boiled down" into useful terms. Two rather coarse-grained issues are: Where is the distribution centered? and How concentrated is it? The first question deals with location, the second with dispersion.

Location

Let us refer this aspect to visual impressions of the histogram. The most conspicuous visual features are usually how many "peaks" there are and where they are located. That value of the random variable (on the baseline)* opposite which a peak occurs is called a *mode*. For that point to qualify as a mode, the number of cases at that point must be much greater than in adjacent classes.

---

*It is a common error to think that it is the peak itself that is the mode. This mistake is like confusing a building with an address.

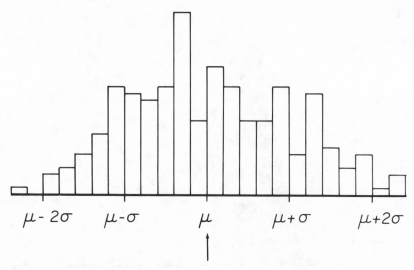

$\mu - 2\sigma$ $\mu - \sigma$ μ $\mu + \sigma$ $\mu + 2\sigma$

Figure 4.6. A histogram of 250 artificial data randomly generated from a Gaussian variate. Note that although there is only one true mode (which would be located at the arrow), there are a number of false modes due to the fluctuations from random sampling.

There may be multiple modes; but unless each mode involves many cases, false modes may readily be created by sampling fluctuations (fig. 4.6). Much fanciful speculation results from overinterpretation of random variation or from some unconscious quirk in the reading or graphing of results. Of all the common measures of location, the mode is the one most at the mercy of sampling fluctuation and of observer bias.

A second index of location (fig. 4.7A) is to think of a histogram as a flat figure to be divided in two parts by one vertical cut. The division point that divides it equally is the *median*. If in turn each part is halved, the new dividing points are the (lower and upper) *quartiles*. And in general, if a cut is made so that the lowest k percent of the distribution lies to the left, the cutting point is the kth *percentile*. Those interested in body height commonly call on a few cardinal percentiles (e.g., 3, 10, 20, etc.) to assess one reading in a single patient. Of course, the individual percentiles depend on the age and sex of the patient. In practice, any particular percentile is found by arranging the sample values in ascending order and finding what percentage of values lie below each point. This representation is the (sample) *cumulative distribution function* (fig. 4.7B). If the sample size is odd, the sample median will be that value at the 50th percentile; if it is even, we average the two central values.

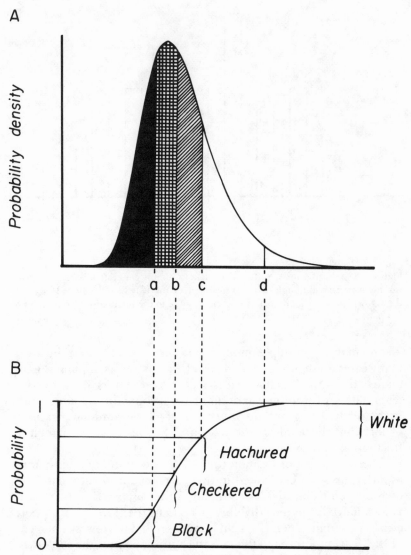

Figure 4.7. Some features of a continuous distribution. *A:* The four areas (*black, checkered, hachured,* and *white*) are equal. Then *b* is the median, or 50th percentile; *a* is the lower quartile, or 25th percentile; *c* is the upper quartile, or 75th percentile; and *d* is the 97th percentile, i.e., 97 percent of the area lies to the left of it and 3 percent to the right. *B:* The cumulative distribution function for the same variate. Against the value of the variate is plotted the probability or area that lies to the left of that point.

A third index of location is to think of the histogram as a sheet of rigid metal cut out exactly to scale and which we wish to balance about a knife edge at right angles to the baseline. The position of the knife edge at which it balances is the *mean*, or the *average*. All readers are familiar with finding averages by adding all the sample values and dividing by the number of sample values. But those with an eye for balance may find it easy enough to guess the mean even if the distribution has a bizarre shape. Note that (unlike the mode) the mean need not equal any actual sample value. When we say that the American family contains on average 1.37 girls and 1.41 boys (or some such figures), we do not expect to see any actual family with that horrifying composition.

Dispersion

The commonest and simplest measure of dispersion of a distribution is the so-called *range*, i.e., the lowest and the highest values observed. This measure is easy to grasp and apply, and for that reason it is commonly recorded in publications of data or of the results of an experiment. It has the disadvantage of being sensitive to sample size. The larger the sample, the more likely it is to include an extreme value. It is the oldest physicians that have the strangest tales to tell. But we do not expect the truth to be affected by experience, merely our knowledge of the truth. A characteristic so dependent on experience is not likely to be a stable descriptor of a population. For this reason it is considered much safer to use measures, the sample values of which bear little *systematic* relationship to the sample size. The experienced and the inexperienced are then concerned with the same problem. But while the estimates themselves will show little systematic relationship to the sample size, the greater the experience, the more precise the estimator of the variation will be.

There are two stable measures of dispersion or scatter in common use. Like the measures of location, they can be applied to any naturally occurring set of measurements the reader is likely to encounter. (By "naturally occurring," I mean the native readings such as will emerge from empirical studies. I make no promises if the reader uses ratios, logarithms, reciprocals, or any other result of the *processing* of the native readings.)

The more noncommittal measure is the difference between two sample percentiles. The most favored pair are the two quartiles (that is, the 25th and the 75th percentiles), and the difference between them is the *interquartile range*. Naturally, the true quartiles encompass the central 50 percent of the distribution (or the sample estimates of the values encompass half of the sample values, as the case may be). Another such measure is the central 95 percent range (commonly, if unhappily, called the "normal range"), i.e., that between the 2.5th and the 97.5th percentiles.

The other approach is usually a more sensitive and balanced measure, which averages how far the observations are from the mean. Unfortunately, if one simply computes the average deviation from the mean (those above the mean being called positive, and those below it negative), the answer will always turn out to be zero whatever the form of the distribution. Such an index that always gives the same answer obviously tells us nothing about the dispersion of the variate. This anomaly is avoided by squaring all the deviations, which makes them positive. The average (found in the usual way) of these squares is called the *variance*. Much of the sting is taken out of the idea of variance when it is seen as nothing more than an average. Since it is, of course, in square measure, most scientists prefer to convert it back into the original scale of measurement by taking the square root of the average (variance), the resulting value being termed the *standard deviation.** Note that if we change the scale of the original measurements, we change the mean and the standard deviation in proportion. For instance, if the average and the standard deviation of the height of American males are 70 and 3 inches respectively, the corresponding values in centimeters would be (70)(2.54) and (3)(2.54), i.e., 177.8 and 7.62 respectively. The variance (being in square measure) would be increased by a factor of $(2.54)^2 = 6.4516$. For height it would be $(6.4516)(3)^2 = 58.0644$.

Descriptors for Other Features of a Distribution
• *In general, a distribution is* not *adequately described by the mean and the standard deviation.*

Two very different distributions may have the same mean; a little thought will make it clear that a distribution and its mirror image will always have the same variance, even if the distribution is highly asymmetrical (fig. 4.8).

There are various ways by which statisticians attempt to describe

---

*Many writers, perhaps because they have misgivings about what the true distribution of results is like, quote the range rather than the standard deviation; but if the distribution is in doubt, the properties of the range are unknown, whereas (as we shall see later in this chapter) we can still make useful inferences from the standard deviation. There is thus all the more reason for furnishing the standard deviation in preference to the range.

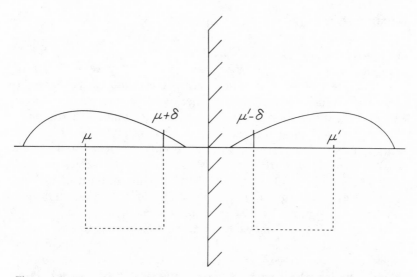

Figure 4.8. The variance of the mirror image (*right*) of a positively skewed distribution (*left*). One typical component is singled out, δ units above the mean (μ); its mirror image is the same distance below the mirror image of the mean (μ'). While the signs of the deviations are different, when squared, they become equal. (The areas represented by the squares in dashed lines are equal.) From symmetry, their probability densities (vertical intercepts) are equal, so the products of the areas of the squares and their probability densities will be equal. The same relationship is true for any point and its mirror image.

asymmetry. These ways are not altogether equivalent, and they vary a good deal in complexity. Visual impressions are mostly based on the relationship of the principal mode to the other features. If most of the distribution and the mean and (naturally) the median lie to the right of the mode, the distribution is *positively skewed* or (more correctly) *skewed to the right*, and conversely.*

Further descriptive features of distributions are more elusive. They may be "flat-topped," i.e., shaped like the profile of a brick; or have a sharp central peak and long tails in both directions, like two ski jumps back to back. The usual standard of reference is the Gaussian, or normal, distribution, which is symmetrical, convex upwards in its central part, and concave upwards in its tails (fig. 4.5C).

*There is a deplorable habit growing up, mainly among biologists, of incorrectly using the expression "skewed to the right" to mean that the sample average value is higher than expected. In that case, the correct term is either "has a systematically greater mean" or "is positively biased," depending on what its origin is.

SOME PROPERTIES OF THE VARIANCE

Independence of Random Variables

When we discussed it above, we perceived independence of events as an absence of any systematic correspondence between the outcomes. *A* has no impact on whether or not *B* occurs if and only if *A* and *B* are independent. Much the same idea may be carried over to random variables; but since a random variable must have not only a probability but (unlike a simple event) a value associated with it as well, we must in this case pay attention to the values.

Yachtsmen are only too well aware that no amount of tacking east and west advances the boat one inch north or south. There is no "rate of exchange" between these movements.

Example 4.10. Two boats are about to start at the same time and place. One is to sail a leg of random length that is either due east or due west of the starting point (we suppose the two are equally likely): the length of such legs is symmetrically distributed about zero on an east-west axis. Thus, treating distance west as negative and east as positive, *on average* (but only on average), the boat will not move from the starting point. The other boat is to follow a similar pattern, but on the north-south axis (fig. 4.9). On average, how far apart will the boats be after each has sailed one leg?

There is little that we gain by examining the averages of the individual legs, for they are both zero. Yet quite obviously the distance between the boats is never negative and will mostly be greater than zero. But if we consider the average of the squares of the distances they travel, we can appeal to the famous theorem that the square of the hypotenuse of a right-angled triangle equals the sum of the squares of the other two sides: the triangle is right-angled because the distances are independent. By definition, the average of the square of the distance of a boat from the starting point is its variance. Thus, the average of the square of the distance between the two boats is the sum of the variances.

I advance this image to coax the reader to accept the following principle (which for the bloodthirsty can be proved with excruciating rigor):

PRINCIPLE 1. *If two random variables are independent, the variance of their sum is the sum of their variances.*

Now consider the special case where the variances for each of the legs sailed by the boats is 8 square miles. The standard deviation for each is the square root of this quantity, or 2.828 . . . miles.

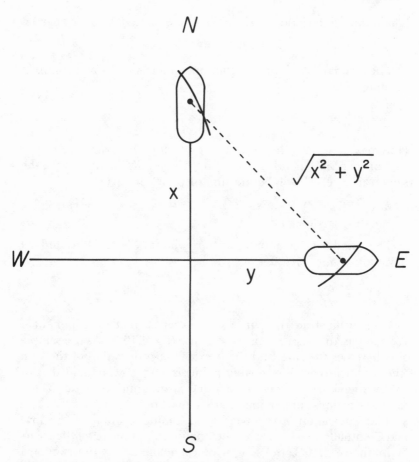

Figure 4.9. Two boats sail a random distance on courses that are at right angles to each other. Their distance apart will be the hypotenuse (the interrupted line) of the right-angled triangle, and hence the square root of the sum of the squares of the two distances sailed.

On average, the square of the distance between the boats will be the sum:

8 + 8 = 16,

of which the square root, 4, is *the standard deviation of their sum.*

If at the end of each leg, the boats sail directly to meet each other, the distance each will have to sail to reach the midpoint between them will be half the total. Thus we find that

The standard deviation of their "sum" (combined distance apart) is

$$\sqrt{8 \times 2} = 4.$$

The standard deviation of their mean distance from a common meeting place is

$$\frac{4}{2} = \sqrt{\frac{8}{2}} = 2.$$

One may generalize this result step by step. The variance of the sum of three independent random variables, X, Y, and Z, with the same variance, σ^2, will be the sum of their variances:

$$\text{var}(X + Y + Z) = \text{var}[(X + Y) + Z] = \text{var}(X + Y) + \text{var}(Z)$$
$$= \text{var}(X) + \text{var}(Y) + \text{var}(Z) = 3\sigma^2$$

The standard deviation *of the sum* will be $\sqrt{3\sigma^2}$. The standard deviation *of the sample average* will be

$$\frac{\sqrt{3\sigma^2}}{3} = \frac{\sigma}{\sqrt{3}}$$

We may illustrate this pattern if we keep each new component at right angles to the previous hypotenuse (fig. 4.10A). As the sample size increases to n, we find that the standard deviation of the sum (the distance from the starting point) is always $\sqrt{n\sigma^2}$ and that of the average is $\sigma/\sqrt{n}$. The former gets larger, but not so fast as the sample size does, and an increasing "snail" results (fig. 4.10B). The standard deviation of the average is forming a diminishing spiral and eventually reaches zero. The relationship is made a little clearer in figure 4.10C, the length of each line being the standard deviation of the sum (σ_T) and that of the segment below the dot being the standard deviation of the mean (σ_M). The ratio between them is equal to the sample size.

The Law of Large Numbers

The reader may wonder why I feel so strongly about these points that I should be prepared to compromise my objective of simplicity. But what we have just found is of the greatest importance.

PRINCIPLE 2. *If we take the* average *of a sample of independent values of the same random variable, its standard deviation gets smaller as the sample gets larger.*

That is, the larger the sample, the more precise the statement we can make about the true value of the mean. If we could get a large

enough sample, the standard deviation, not of the individual readings, but *of the average* would become zero, and we would know the
mean exactly.

This principle, commonly called "the law of averages" by the
laity, is one of the Laws of Large Numbers. It tells us how fast (with
respect to sample size) the precision improves. It also points out
that if the variance of the initial variate is small, the same degree of
assurance can be attained with a smaller sample, and vice versa.

But this law also corrects what is a common mistake. Many people talk loosely about random effects "canceling out." This notion
is quite false. Random effects do not cancel out. We cannot argue
that Democratic votes cancel with Republican votes and that the
bigger the electorate the more predictable the plurality. Other
things being equal, the bigger the electorate, the *more* variable the
margin of victory will be in *absolute* numbers; but the *less* variable
when expressed in *percentages*.

It also helps us to maintain perspective about the conclusions
that one may draw from data. This topic suffers from two kinds of
extremists. The one is forever loudly declaiming "You can tell
nothing from one case." This heresy I have elsewhere (12) called
the snobbery of large numbers. The other enthusiast, because he is
using a method that is ten times as precise as any previous one,
smugly claims the right to overtrump all previous accumulated
experience by a few privileged observations. The variances of the
means tell us how to strike a balance among these rival claims and
how to weigh conflicting evidence on its merits.

THE GAUSSIAN DISTRIBUTION

The variance of a random variable is a mean. It is the mean of
the squares of all the individual deviations from the mean. In the
preceding section we saw that the more data are added, the greater
the variance of the sum. For independent data, this increase is
more than offset by averaging, so that *the variance of the mean* steadily falls with the increasing size of the sample. If we took the cubes
(or any higher power) of the deviations, averaged them, and then
took the corresponding root, increasing the size of sample would
damp down the rate of increase even faster. So while I shall not
attempt to show it formally, the reader will not be surprised to
learn that the only features of importance for the distribution of
the mean of a large sample are the mean and (to a lesser extent) the
variance. Other averages eventually become negligible. The distribution that is identified by the mean and the variance alone and

to which all other features are irrelevant is the Gaussian (fig. 4.5C). It is often called by the misleading name "normal."
• *The term* normal distribution *has nothing to do with normality in the clinical, the esthetic, the moral, or any other sense.*

Indeed, the Gaussian distribution fits comparatively few histograms of biological data.

The main virtue of this distribution is that (for the reasons just given) it is a surprisingly good descriptor of *the distribution of the mean of a large sample.* It is vital to know what this statement means.

Example 4.11. Individual readings of blood urea nitrogen (BUN) on specimens from independent individuals selected from the population at large do *not* follow the Gaussian distribution. If I take the

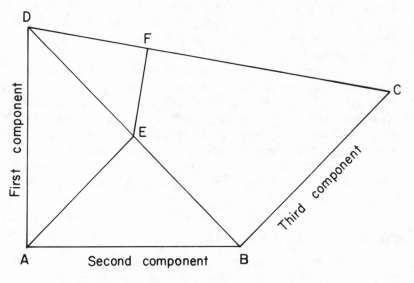

A

Figure 4.10. The snails of uncertainty. *A:* The first two components, *DA* and *AB*, represent the standard deviations of the first two data values. They are shown at right angles because they are independent. The standard deviation of their sum is *DB*, the hypotenuse. The third, similar component, *BC*, is at right angles to that hypotenuse, and the new hypotenuse, *CD*, is the standard deviation of the sum of three sample values. But *DE*, which is half the length of *DB*, is the standard deviation of the *average* of the first two; and *DF*, which is one third of the length of *DC*, is the standard deviation of the average of the first three. *B:* An extension of the process to the first 25 sample values. The standard deviations of the sum (σ_T) and of the mean (σ_M) for each step are represented by the distances from the center of the two snails. The former expands with decreasing speed; the latter contracts. *C:* Comparison of σ_T and σ_M, according to sample size. The ratio between them is the sample size, and their product is a constant, the variance of a single component.

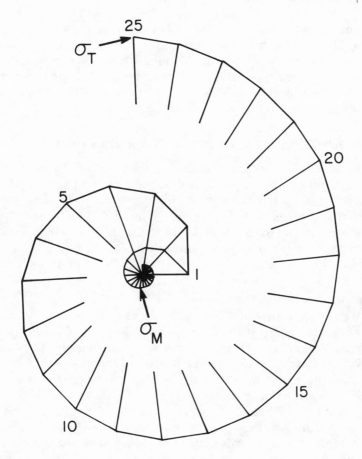

B

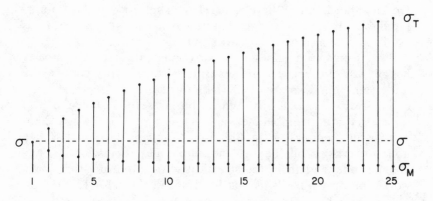

C

mean of the values from 100 such subjects, I have one sample mean. If I average a further 100 readings, I have a second sample mean. If I repeat this process 500 times, I have 500 sample means, each from an independent sample of 100 subjects. The histogram of these 500 mean values may be expected to follow a Gaussian distribution fairly closely.

INDEPENDENCE, REGRESSION, AND CORRELATION

It will be clear from the foregoing that a full description of a distribution may be simple; it may also be very complicated. In the latter case, we often make use of what are coarse all-purpose descriptors, the mean, the mode, etc. When we come to treat two random variables together (as height and weight, or blood pressure and age), we must make statements not only about each member of the pair but also about whether they are *independent* or not.

Independence

We have already had a notional explanation of the latter term: *A* is independent of *B* if *B* tells us nothing about *A*, and conversely.

Example 4.12. If we want to guess what a human male's systolic blood pressure (in mm Hg—millimeters of mercury) may be and we have no data whatsoever on him, we may argue that it will scarcely be below 50 or above 300. The best guess—a blind guess— is perhaps 140. Needless to say, it would have no great claims to accuracy. Now we can improve this guess by knowing his age. For a child of three months, this figure would be exceptionally high; for a man age seventy, it would be unusually low. Then since age changes our guess, age and blood pressure are not independent. On the other hand, if there is no relationship between the hour of the day at which he was born and his blood pressure when he is aged forty, then the variates are (mutually) independent.

That seems clear enough. Unfortunately, the term *independent* has all sorts of other meanings outside statistics, which confuse the understanding. Two are of special importance.

The word *independent* is used (in business, for instance) of two things that are incompatible with each other. "The Brown Company is independent of the Robinson Company" means that they do not overlap at all. That relationship makes them *disjoint*. They are not independent in the statistical sense. Knowing that Jones works for Brown's tells us that he is not working for Robinson's.

Example 4.13. Since an adult cannot at the same time be both a dwarf (i.e., with height less than, say, 150 cm) and a giant (with a

height over 210 cm), these states are disjoint; they are not indepen-
dent. Being a giant is certainly not independent of being a dwarf.
As near as makes no difference:
• *Mutually exclusive events are never independent.*

The other main confusion arises from the terms one uses when
plotting a graph. How much income tax a man must pay may be
plotted as a function of his income. Ordinarily, we would call the
income tax "the dependent variable" and the income "the independent variable." But this usage has nothing to do with statistical
independence. Indeed, since by knowing the one we can calculate
the other, neither is independent of the other. Note a further
point.
• *Statistical independence is a* mutual relationship between random
variables or events.

Regression

It is meaningless to talk about statistical independence if either
of the quantities is nonrandom.

Example 4.14. Suppose a pharmacologist is trying out the effects
of various dosages of a new drug on intestinal motility. He is plan-
ning to give the next three patients the systematically varied doses
10 mg two, three, and four times a day respectively. Then the dose
is varying mathematically, but it is not varying randomly. He may
show a relationship between dosage and effect. Such a relationship
is known as a *regression;* the cause (dosage) is called the *regressor
variable,* and the effect is the *response variable.* Dosage and effect
might prove to be nonindependent if he were to make dosage
random; but he did not do so in this experiment, and the term
statistical dependence or *independence* does not have any meaning in
this case.

It is usually not possible by statistical means, without appealing
to other sources of information, to show whether or not two random variables are independent. One of these sources is conceptual
unrelatedness. If we are satisfied that two things are unrelated, that
*we can find, devise, or imagine no connection between them, however
remote,* then we may regard them as notionally independent. However, the condition stated in italics is a severe one, and not lightly
invoked; and even so, it is not a statistical statement.* Another
source is to appeal to the known, or inferred, distribution of the

---

*There are special circumstances in which two events cannot, for formal reasons,
be independent. It is thus wise to regard notional and formal dependence as analogous rather than interchangeable terms.

data. One outstanding example is the Gaussian distribution. Leaving aside bizarre exceptions (30), one may argue that if two Gaussian variates are uncorrelated (see below), they are independent.

In general, however, it is difficult to demonstrate that two variables with unspecified distributions are independent; instead, we have to make do with a coarser yardstick (just as the mode or the variance is a coarse yardstick that tells us only so much about a distribution).

Correlation

At this point we shall not even attempt to deal with covariance formally. It suffices to say that it is something like variance that measures how closely pairs of readings (say height and weight on the same subject) stick together when there is variation among subjects. (The variance of a single variable can, in fact, be seen as the covariance of the variate with itself.) The easiest (and still the best) way to get a feel for covariance is to construct a *scatter diagram.* Each *pair* of values is plotted as a point, its abscissa being one variate and its ordinate the other. Inspecting the diagram may suggest a pattern. If the points make a more or less elliptical cluster, one tries to fit a straight line convincingly through the thick of the points, parallel to the longer axis of the ellipse. If this line is neither horizontal nor vertical, we suspect that the variates are correlated. The more elongated the ellipse, the closer the correlation. There may be a few wild points, but one's assessment of direction should not be unduly swayed by them.

When we want to grapple with this relationship quantitatively, we find that the measurement of covariance depends on scale. The covariance between height in centimeters and weight in grams will be greater than that between height in inches and weight in ounces. To avoid this irrelevancy, it is customary to rescale the data in such a way as to make the index of relatedness the same whatever the units of measurement. The resulting measure is known as the *correlation coefficient.* Various examples are given in figure 4.11. The highest possible value it may take is 1 (the perfect correlation, which means that all the points in the scatter diagram will fall on a line with a positive slope). A value of -1 (the minimum possible) means the same, but with a negative slope. A value of 0 means that the variables are uncorrelated. A significant correlation (i.e., one not readily ascribable to the chance results of random sampling) is always evidence of nonindependence. But the fact that the correlation coefficient is 0 is only weak evidence that they are independent—certainly not proof.

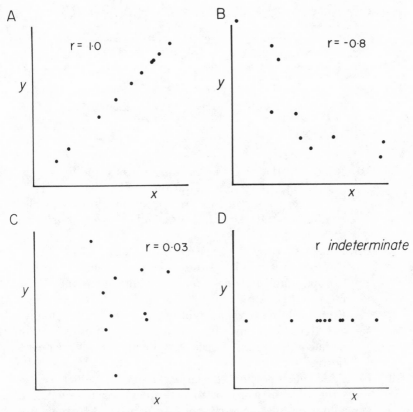

Figure 4.11. Scatter diagrams and correlation coefficients. The coordinates of each point correspond to the values of the two random variables that characterize it. *A:* All the points lie on a straight line with a positive slope, and the correlation coefficient is unity. *B:* There is some scatter, and the main axis has a negative slope. *C:* The two variables are close to being uncorrelated, and there is no clear main axis. *D:* All the points lie on a straight line, and one might expect the correlation coefficient to be unity, as in *A*. However, the ordinates of all the points are equal, and it is not clear that the quantity represented on it is variable (let alone a random variable). Hence, the correlation coefficient would be meaningless, and the formal calculations show that it equals 0/0, which is indeterminate.

PROBLEMS

4.1. "It is the oldest physicians that have the strangest tales to tell." Consider *all* the reasons why this statement is likely to be true.

4.2. The data in table 4.1 on birth weights in Moroccan Jewish babies in Tel Aviv were published by Fried and Davies (31).

    a. Find the sample range and median.

Table 4.1. Birth Weight in Kilograms of Moroccan Jewish Babies Born in Tel Aviv

3.32	3.45	3.30	3.70	4.25	3.50	3.85	2.80	2.60
4.05	3.00	3.50	3.35	3.75	3.75	2.80	3.48	2.77
3.58	3.26	3.40	3.70	3.12	2.50	3.55	3.70	3.32
3.25	3.46	2.95	3.15	3.45	3.42	3.74	3.55	3.65
3.80	4.05	3.45	3.35	2.82	3.70	3.27	3.25	3.50
3.35	3.70	3.06	3.10	3.20	3.45	3.30	4.10	3.52

Source: Data of Fried and Davies (31).

    b. Represent the data as a histogram using the groupings 2.6–2.79, 2.8–2.99, etc. Find the mode.

    c. Repeat *b*, combining the first two categories and also combining the last two. (Remember: *area* represents *probability*.)

    d. Repeat *b*, using the groupings 2.5–2.69, 2.7–2.79, etc. Compare the results of these two groupings.

    e. Compare and comment on the values of the mean, the mode, and the median.

    f. From each of the values subtract the sample mean to give the deviation, carefully distinguishing positive from negative deviations. Verify that the average of the deviations is zero.

4.3. Consider the following spacial arrangement, which represents the plan of a group of seventeen apartments. Each symbol represents an apartment. Those marked *D* are damp; the rest are normal. The neighbors note that the affected apartments are in a straight line and suspect that the dampness is due to a defective drain.

```
        D N N N
        N D N
  N     N N D
  N     N
  N N N N
```

    a. What is the probability that three of the apartments picked at random would lie in a straight line? (The number of possible different ways in which three things can be picked from 17 is $(17.16.15)/(3.2.1) = 680$.)

    b. What else would a probabilist take into consideration in examining the drain theory?

4.4. The following four letters are found in random order: O, P, S, and T. Theory shows that they can be arranged in twenty-four distinct ways.

a. What are these twenty-four ways?

b. What is the probability that they are intended to be used to represent an English word?

c. *If* it is English, what is the conditional probability that the word is STOP?

d. Would the answer to *c* be changed by the color of the letters or the place where the letters were found?

4.5. Consider the role of independence in the help given by the hints in each of the following cases.

a. What is the tallest mountain in the world? (Hint: Annapurna is 26,503 feet high.)

b. Is a spider an insect? (Hint: Insects have six legs.)

c. Which of the Bachs invented sonata form? (Hint: The battle of Tagliacozzo took place in 1268.)

d. What is the height of the tallest mountain in the world? (Hint: Annapurna is 26,503 feet high.)

4.6. What is the impact of knowledge on freedom? Does it enhance it? If so, how? If not, is loss of freedom a fair price for enlightenment? Are there other possible answers? Can the form of the question be usefully recast?

5 | Statistical Inference

Probability algebra is part of mathematics. Like much of pure mathematics it deals with the formal exploration of possible systems.

Statistics is a branch of science. Like most of science, it deals with the world of actual experience.

There are probabilists who become bookmakers, but they are atypical. Likewise, there are many highly theoretical statisticians who never look at data; but they are ultimately concerned with the theory of extracting information from empirical data (that is, data obtained by actual observation and experimentation).

Statistical methods are widely used in biology and (not to mince words) widely misused. A brief synopsis of methods is given in the appendix; but those who do not care to read it will be at no disadvantage in reading this book. My experience is that mistakes in statistical analysis involves (in order of increasing importance): (1) the calculations; (2) the areas of application; (3) the interpretation.

Let us discuss them one at a time.

ERRORS OF CALCULATION

These errors are purely technical, and in principle are readily avoidable. The main preventive measure is care: checking and rechecking the calculations and the reasoning to make sure that no errors have been made and perpetuated. This topic will not have much importance to the kind of reader I have in mind, who is unlikely to be processing data; so I shall not labor it.

A second valuable method, and one which the discerning reader will wish to know, involves a simple list of certainties and impossibilities that may be used as checks. Thus, for sample values from any data whatsoever, the following statements must be true.

1. The sample mean must be greater than the smallest, and less than the largest, sample value. If the sample range of values is quoted, the sample mean must lie within it. (These inequalities strictly apply to all except the trivial case where the data values are all equal.)
2. The standard deviation and the variance, or any sum of squares, will be rarely zero and never negative.
3. It is impossible for *all* the sample results to lie less, or *all* to lie more, than one sample standard deviation from the sample mean.
4. Neither the true, nor the sample, correlation coefficient can be less than -1 or greater than $+1$.

These statements are given here for reference; but readers may already be familiar with some or all of them.

Finally, there is common sense. Is the answer repugnant? This criterion is not to be used to make final judgments. But it should give warning: to go back yet once again over the data, the calculations, and the reasoning. Nevertheless, when one finally casts a conclusion aside, it should not be on grounds of common sense alone. Indeed, I suspect that nobody with that rare commodity, true common sense, would ever suppose otherwise.

ERRORS OF APPLICATION

Every statistical procedure is based on certain assumptions; and it is part of the responsibility of the statistician to verify these assumptions in each set of data to which he applies that test. This demand is obvious, and in principle well-known; but it is surprising how often even statisticians in their papers make no statement that they have, in fact, verified these assumptions. No doubt they have paid due attention to them and suppose it is superfluous to mention the fact. But a critical reader will be cautious about taking any such step for granted; and this caution is especially wise if there are any signs that the writer does not have some expert knowledge of statistics. For this reason it is always prudent for the writer to discuss the assumptions explicitly and (so far as editorial policy allows) to publish the data as fully as possible. At times the writer or the reviewer of the manuscript should, for good reason, apply pressure upon the editor to allow space for these inclusions.

Sometimes the assumptions are very *weak,* or undemanding: they suppose little that anybody would really doubt in the particular case. For instance, the assumption may be that height is (at least in principle) on a continuous scale of measurement; or that all patients are either living or dead. Sometimes, however, the assumptions are *strong,* or exacting. Thus, a great body of analysis is based on the assumption that data follow the Gaussian ("normal") distribution, or that they are mutually independent, and that they come from the same population or from populations with the same mean and variance. In data that have been collected and presented, any or all of these assumptions may be not even approximately true.

According to what may be assumed, the statistician has his choice among tests. The so-called *nonparametric* tests* call for a minimum of assumptions. Other tests are exquisitely dependent on the assumptions. The latter include tests on higher moments and, in particular, tests on variances (notably Bartlett's test for equality of variance).

A third group of tests occupy a peculiar intermediate position. Strictly speaking, they are based on arguments from very precise and restricted assumptions. But under certain favorable conditions at least, the tests (for what they are designed to do) are surprisingly little affected by even quite serious departures from the assumptions. Such procedures are said to be *robust.*

The most famous and widely invoked example of robustness (mentioned in chapter 4) is that if we take the average (or sum) of a reasonably sized sample of values selected randomly and independently from almost any single distribution, a priori this mean will have a distribution that is close to Gaussian ("normal"). This result is so important that it merits a good deal of clarifying discussion. Note the following points.

The Property Is Corporate, Not Individual

This result is a statement about averages of many readings, not about the individual readings themselves. We may use it in making statements

---

*Some of the common nonparametric tests the reader may meet are the binomial and chi-square tests; the Mann-Whitney, or Wilcoxon, or *U* test; the Kolmogorov-Smirnov test; the Spearman and the Kendall rank correlation tests; the Kruskal-Wallis and Friedman tests for the analysis of variance. It may be worthwhile to know these names, because they crop up from time to time in scientific papers and it is helpful to know what their broad theoretical standings are. But I do not propose to say anything further about them.

about groups, e.g., whether men are on the average taller than women; or professors on the average heavier than bus drivers. But it does not apply to individual readings.

Example 5.1. It is often necessary to obtain a test measurement in order to decide whether an individual person has a disease. The test is used to distinguish or *discriminate* between a sick person and a well person. But an individual person is not a large sample, and there is no point in arguing from the theorems that refer to large samples. If in such cases one wishes to appeal to the properties of the Gaussian distribution, then it is necessary that the individual observations should themselves follow this distribution.*

What do we mean by saying that a probability is a priori? After the sample average has been calculated, it will be a perfectly definite quantity, not a random variable, and hence it has no distribution, any more than Abraham Lincoln's height had a distribution. To say that a variate has a near-Gaussian distribution has meaning only while it remains a prediction. A pragmatic test of that statement would be that if we were to collect a very large number of such samples, compute the mean for each, and make a histogram of these means, it would have an approximately Gaussian form. Of course, we do not have any such pragmatic method of demonstration when we are applying the theorem to only one set of results.

The Property Applies to Sums Only

For the generalization to apply, the data values must be *added*, not put together in some other way.

Example 5.2. Where the measurements are *multiplied* together (as often happens in chemical reactions or the dynamics of enzyme pathways), their product will not approximate the Gaussian form.

The Sample Must Be of Reasonable Size

In general I suggest that the issues are (a) Whether the distribution of *individual* values is symmetrical or not. For symmetrical distributions this law of the distribution of means may be invoked for smaller sizes of sample than for asymmetrical ones. (b) The general form of the parent distribution. The mean for a sample from even the square-topped (the so-called rectangular) distribution is barely distinguishable from the Gaussian if the sample size is twenty or greater. If there is a single central mode, a small sample would suffice. On the other hand a U-shaped distribution (one with

---

*Sometimes it is possible by special methods to make non-Gaussian data into Gaussian form; but that is a more complicated matter.

modes at both extremes), even if symmetrical, would approach the Gaussian much more slowly, and it might be wise to use the law of the means only if the sample size is perhaps one-hundred or greater in such cases. However, there is no magical size that will allay all our troubles, and in general, the bigger the sample, the more accurate the approximation.

The Scope of the Approximation Varies

In most practical situations I know of, the results of this approximation are most accurate towards the center and least accurate in the tails. They should therefore be applied with caution to extreme values.

ERRORS OF INTERPRETATION

My concern here is with what meaning a statistical result has as evidence. It is still embarrassingly common for a writer to carry an analysis through flawlessly, and in discussing his findings, to misrepresent seriously what the analysis means.

Sometimes this misrepresentation is purely verbal. Writers refer to *incidence* (which is a rate) when they mean *prevalence* (which is a proportion). They use *skewed* (which is concerned with symmetry) when they mean *biased* (which refers to representativeness). They say *accuracy* (which measures unbiasedness) when they mean *precision* (which is a gauge of reproducibility). They use *parameter* (which is a constant) when they are dealing with a *random variable* or *variate* (which is, naturally, variable). The only remedy for such errors is to recognize that technical vocabulary is tolerable only because it conveys exact meaning. Otherwise, it is a mere vulgarity.
• *No writer or scientist should use a technical word unless prepared, if challenged, to give a correct formal definition of it.*

Indeed, this is a sound principle for all writing whatsoever. I hope the reader will cultivate a thoroughly merciless witchhunt for such lapses in scholarly writings, especially those of the august, which tend to be imitated. In the Glossary I furnish a brief vocabulary that would enable critical readers to do so.

Nevertheless, though the fact is often regrettable, technical vocabulary must in some degree be mutable: partly because the number of new ideas constantly strains the existing vocabulary, and lay words such as *likelihood* and *hazard* then have to be appropriated for technical use; and partly because as ideas evolve, the original meaning has proved too restrictive (e.g., *pain*) or corresponds to a false notion (e.g., *hysteria*, which originally ascribed the symptoms to disorder of the uterus; or *melancholia*, which was thought due to blackness of the bile). So long as a writer defines any special meaning that he ascribes to a word, he is still within his rights; but such artificialities should be used sparingly.

Reasoning is a sterner master. Those adventurous enough may define and defend their own pattern of reasoning; but writers that *borrow a standard procedure* on the warrant of some expert have no choices about what the conclusions mean. None. This warning will be amply illustrated in the next chapter in the context of testing hypotheses.

THE SCOPE OF STATISTICS

There are three main activities in which the statistician proper engages: estimation; testing hypotheses; and making decisions. Each has its legitimate area of use; but much damage results from confusion among these uses. Surprisingly often, investigators become involved in testing hypotheses when they would do better to be engaged in estimation. What is worse, granting agencies laying down guidelines for applications confuse the activities; they may require a statement of a hypothesis in every application, even in the case of research that has nothing to do with a hypothesis and which could not be usefully dealt with by testing one. There is the implication that anything that is not exploring a hypothesis is not science. But this supposition is manifestly absurd. Determining the tertiary structure of growth hormone does not center strategically on any hypothesis at all. (Of course, in exploring such a problem, one may develop hundreds of tactical hypotheses at intermediate stages; but they are not such as can be stated in advance as a strategic hypothesis.) An enquiry into the relationship of height to age may well be an exercise in pure estimation. Finding an optimal critical level of blood pressure at which treatment should be instituted involves values and costs and cannot be dealt with by either estimation or testing a hypothesis. Other instances will occur in what follows.

It is not the purpose of this book to confront the technical details of these topics. But I shall try to give some insight into the objectives and implication. In the remainder of this chapter we shall consider estimation; and in chapter 6 we shall deal with the other two topics.

ESTIMATION

There are some quantities of scientific importance that may be arrived at by pure deduction. To be sure, they all ultimately depend on some assumptions about what the nature of the physical world is. One might wonder whether or not Euclidean geometry applies to the actual universe we live in; but no serious scientist would think that we should try to determine the logarithms of natural numbers by experimental means.

In contrast, we have the quantities that must be found empirically, that is, by experiment and observation. Those who use the methods are at the mercy of their properties, which are of varying refinement and which they will employ with variable and fallible skill. A concern of the scientist given some imperfect data will be how to extract from it the best information about the measurement of interest. As discussed elsewhere in this book, there may be several different types of limitation on the nicety of the answer.

First, the lack of refinement of an enquiry may be conceptual: the original question may simply have been too vague to allow a precise answer.

Example 5.3. The question "How high is Mount Everest?" is of this type. Does it mean the height of the rock of the mountain? That might be difficult to observe. Does it mean the height of the mountain together with the snow on it? If so, the answer will vary according to the amount of snow (which depends on the season). Does it refer to the average height of the mountain? If so, above what? If the sea, is it at high tide, or what? Those of us solemnly filling in our weights on our passports must wonder under what conditions one is recording the correct weight: before or after breakfast? There is no remedy here but to recognize the limitations of the question and, if necessary, to clarify it.

Then second, the uncertainty may be dominated by the limitations of the apparatus. Sometimes the issue may be one of calibration.

Example 5.4. Properly specified, the length of a bone on X-ray is a sufficiently definite quantity to admit of a refined answer; but not if one has only a coarsely calibrated yardstick, or a scale made of wood (which is perhaps warped) to measure it with.

Sometimes there are intrinsic physical limits.

Example 5.5. One cannot measure any temperature above the melting point of glass with a glass thermometer. I doubt that a psychometrist can devise a convincing measure of the intelligence of a subject more intelligent than the psychometrist.

The issue in these cases is one of resolving power; and the only prospect here is to change the properties of the instrument, or to devise a new approach.

Then third, the defects may be genuine random variation; and the remedy is then estimation, which we shall now discuss.

ESTIMATES AND ESTIMATORS

Estimation deals with the question of how we can form a best *estimate*—a guess, but an educated guess—of some quantity, when the only observations of it that we can make are flawed somewhat by random error. It comes as no great surprise, perhaps, that there are many possible *estimators,** that is, recipes for finding answers, no one of which has unique status. There are some seven or eight common estimators contending; but there are a great many others developed for particular, even unique, problems. What answer should be given, in general, depends on three factors: what is known, or may be assumed, about the system; what properties we wish the answer to have; and how much effort and expertise is available for using the estimator. Let us take them one by one.

Prior Knowledge

Here we have to be concerned with two components of knowledge. One is knowledge about the process itself and how we might expect the distribution to behave. The other is knowledge about what the values of the parameters are that characterize the distribution.

The Nature of the Process. There is some risk that the habits of dealing with data may become ingrained; as a result, one loses insight into their arbitrary character to the point at which even the obvious may be obscured. The most insidious of these beliefs is that the main thing to know about a distribution is the average. This is so often a sound claim that one may find it hard to think in other terms, unless one's native wit has not been sullied by education. Let us consider some examples.

Example 5.6. Suppose that a gastroenterologist is trying to find out what the size of a gallstone is in a particular patient. Casual examination of the X-rays and his experience might suggest to him that it is roughly egg-shaped. From the point of view of removing

*The distinction between the terms is that an estimator is a plan of analysis; an estimate is a result from one. An estimator is (as it were) a recipe for making a cake, an estimate is a cake. An estimator behaves like a random variable and has a mean, variance, distribution, etc.; it may be biased, efficient, etc. An estimate, on the other hand, is a simple quantity.

it, it may be characterized entirely by finding its largest diameter and its smallest. Let us say that he has ten X-ray images to look at, which were taken from diverse viewpoints that he is prepared to regard as random. How can he best find these two key measurements? The simplest answer is to measure each of the films with one thought in mind: that he wants to find the biggest diameter in any film, and the smallest. There is nothing to be said for taking the average or the variance of the measurements. More generally, if the goal is to find the range of any set of values, all the secure pertinent information is contained in the smallest and the largest values. If one is confident of the mathematical form of the gallstone (for instance, that it is an ellipsoid), there is more information to be coaxed out of the data than taking the extreme measurements. But this latter claim is not always true. In certain cases (the rectangular or uniform distribution), it is again the extreme values that contain all the information, not the average or any other statistical index. For instance, in trying to decide whether a car will fit into a rectangular garage, it is the greatest length, breadth, and height that matter, and no further information is worth having.

Example 5.7. How do we decide if a patient with heart failure is receiving enough oxygen? Obviously, the critical answer does not depend on the mean. If the patient receives twice as much as he needs for ten minutes and during the next ten minutes he then gets none at all, the average will be adequate, but the patient will be dead. Here it is the extreme variation that matters, not the average variation.

Example 5.8. How do we decide how many chromosomes are present in a karyotype? The obvious answer is to count them; but it takes some practice to do so without getting confused and counting the same one twice. The first count shows 44; the second, 45. What does the cytogeneticist do? He might average the result, but an answer of 44.5 would be meaningless. So he counts them a third time, and the answer is 45. Now what does he do? The new average, 44.67, is as meaningless as before. The answer *must be a whole number.* He might take the answer as 45; or he might count it yet once again; and if he is fanatical about it, he may count it several more times. But the answer, when he gets there, shall be a whole number, and the sensible figure to use is the answer that occurs most commonly in his trial counts, not the mean, but the mode. In the same way, an accountant checking a balance will aim for two or more totals that agree, rather than the average of all the calculations.

Prior Knowledge of the Parameters. The investigator is not necessarily the first person to have measured the quantity that he is interested in. There may be a considerable amount of data on the subject already. Why, then, is he collecting more data? Commonly it is because he has misgivings that the published information is applicable to his population of reference. Perhaps he suspects that because of skin pigment, the Negro population he is studying will have a lower rate of skin cancer. But if he found that the frequency differed by a factor of fifty, he would be suspicious that the estimate was not correct. Such a big risk ratio is most unusual in population studies. Hence, he is appealing to prior knowledge at two levels: prior knowledge of the frequency of the disorder and prior knowledge of risk ratios.

Of course, capitalizing on such prior information (what is broadly called "Bayesian estimation") is not mainly a matter of diffuse anxiety. One must at some stage have the courage to say flatly that the findings in this study are at variance with the findings of other writers studying other populations. But while we cannot go into detail about how it is done, there do exist Bayesian methods of toning down the impact of the information in new data. They have been developed and applied in actual problems. We shall have something more to say about them in the next chapter.

Properties of the Estimator

An estimator is something like a method of making a map of the world, or a diagram of the curved surface of the brain. In a map one is trying to represent in two dimensions something that exists in three. Mapping aims at conserving particular properties at the cost of some distortions that destroy other properties: one preserves directions, perhaps, by distorting the uniformity of the scale. In estimation one is trying to boil down a set of exact data into a smaller number of key quantities; and again, one may not be able to preserve all the properties one would like in the answer. In order to make an assessment of a method, one must give some thought to general properties. There is no single yardstick; and the various demands we make may be in more or less open conflict. Some of them are general attributes of the estimator, and apply to samples of any size (unbiasedness, reproducibility, sufficiency, exact distribution) and some, the asymptotic properties, only emerge when the sample size is large (consistency, efficiency, asymptotic distribution). It is worthwhile to devote a little space to each, not for detail, but in order to get some sense of what the issues are and to have some insight into the statistician's problems. The main interest for the general reader is that there are merits in some estimators and demerits in all; and since there is no "metastatistics" that tells us which properties we should prize most and how much, we are well on the way to understanding why statistics remains an art and is not an ironclad discipline.

General Properties

Unbiasedness. An estimator is unbiased if *on average* it gives the right answer. The simple averages worked out by baseball fans are unbiased estimators of the quantity they are measuring.* Of course unbiasedness is not a property of an estimate (i.e., an actual result), merely of an estimator.

Reproducibility. This informal term is usually applied to measurements of an individual quantity. The smaller the variation, the more reproducible. When applied to an estimator, it is gauged by the variance. While this quality is admirable, it is not overriding. One could have an estimator that was reproducibly wrong. To take an absurd extreme, when estimating the mean, if instead of dividing the sum of the data values by the size of the sample, we were to divide by infinity, the answer would always be exactly the same, zero. Nothing could be more reproducible than that; but it would be a useless estimator, since the answer would in no way reflect the data.

Sufficiency. There are elaborate mathematical statements of what this property is. Roughly speaking, a sample statistic is sufficient for a parameter if it embodies all the information about it contained in the sample. It is like a superior lemon squeezer that extracts the last drop of juice and nothing else out of the lemon. I say "and nothing else," for the original sample of data themselves (naturally) contain all the information in that sample. However, one needs a distillate to work with. Strictly, we do not speak of a sufficient estimator, but of one based on a sufficient statistic. Common examples of sufficient statistics include the sample mean and variance of a Gaussian variate which contain all the information in the sample about the true mean and variance respectively.

Tractability. The *Exact Distribution* of a sample estimate is often very complicated. Some estimators (notably the Gaussian) are easier to handle than others.

---

*In contrast, the batting average in cricket is not. It is computed as the number of runs a player scored divided by the number of times he was put out (*not* the number of times he batted). The sample average might be infinite, so the population average cannot be said to exist. In 1953 the Australian Test cricketer, W. A. Johnston, was actually put out only once in eighteen innings and his batting average was 102, although his best friends would not boast that he was a batsman of distinction. With luck in the eighteenth innings, his average would have been infinite.

Large-Sample Properties

Though these properties are capable of precise mathematical treatment, they are not always easy to deal with in practice. The big difficulty is to decide whether the sample is large enough to invoke them.

Consistency. Roughly, this term denotes the property that the estimator is almost sure to get the right answer when the sample is large enough. An estimate untrustworthy for small samples may work well in large ones. The main importance of the term to readers of this book is that it should not be used in the sense of *unvarying* ("The patient's IQ is consistently between 70 and 75") or of *reliable* ("The blood sugar is consistently raised in diabetes").

Efficiency. This is another easily misunderstood term. It has nothing to do with how easy the estimator is to apply. It is a measure of the variance of one estimator as compared with that of competitors. There is a theoretical limit to the efficiency of most estimators, and if this limit ("the lower bound") is attained, the estimator (if consistent) is said to be *absolutely efficient.*

Asymptotic Distribution. Many estimators based on large samples more or less follow the Gaussian distribution. This property is valuable in constructing approximate confidence limits (which we shall discuss shortly).

Feasible Effort and Available Skill

Finally, one must consider whether using the estimator is practicable. An estimator may have excellent properties; but it is apt to be neglected if it is either very tedious to use or so complicated that only very sophisticated readers will understand what is being done and why. On the one hand, we have Haldane's comment (32) about analyzing a study painstakingly carried out over three years by Sjøgren that "an expenditure of 3 hours on calculations concerning it is not excessive." On the other hand, we meet the common attitude of suspicion towards arcane analyses and a great reluctance among even quite sophisticated scientists to use them.

Moreover, one should recognize that even professional analysts are often slow to use procedures that call for very elaborate analysis. Methods that in principle have been devised and are fully warranted, collect dust on the shelf. I have occasionally had to use methods, long described in the literature, that none of my colleagues, however senior, has any actual experience of doing; and none could offer me any guidance.

One may perhaps take into consideration the nature of the data. To use a simple estimator with an efficiency of sixty percent instead of a complicated one with an efficiency of 100 percent is equivalent to randomly discarding 40 percent of the data. How would the person who had gathered the data feel about that? If the data are very difficult to obtain or if (for ethical or other reasons) no further data will be available, one should not spare any effort to coax the last little bit of information from them. If further information is easily to be had and in due course will certainly be available, one may be forgiven for short-circuiting some of the more tedious problems of analysis.

So far we have been thinking about estimators and their properties. What they will, in general, furnish are particular estimates of the parameters of interest. But the thoughtful reader will not be content to be told, for instance, that the number of genes coding for skin color is estimated to be 6. For an estimate is a guess; and the immediate question that it provokes is how good the guess is. It would be comforting to know that the true answer is almost certainly between 5 and 8, but unsettling to find that it is between 2 and 120. A *point estimate* is better than nothing; but the circumspect will want an *interval estimate* as well. A major difficulty is that interval estimates, which furnish some sense of the uncertainty of the estimate, are not even certain estimates of uncertainty. I conclude with one of the common devices for expressing the state of conviction.

CONFIDENCE LIMITS

A topic of special interest is confidence limits. I am not concerned with technical details, which vary according to the problem involved. But a clear understanding of what confidence limits signify is of the utmost importance. There are many misconceptions about them; and on the principle that prevention is better than cure, I propose to try to dispel them first.

In the first place, confidence limits arise in connection with estimation. *They have nothing to do with testing hypotheses.* (See chapter 6.) One still comes across loose statements such as "A test was done at the 95 percent level of confidence." They have no technical meaning at all. They conjure up visions of nervous investigators fortifying themselves with 95 proof whiskey until they have confidence enough to do the test.

Second, *confidence limits are not probability statements about the parameter.* To say that 95 percent confidence limits on the mean of a distribution of uric acid levels are 3 and 5 mg/dl does *not* mean that the probability that the true value lies within these limits is 95 percent. The whole enquiry takes for granted that a true mean exists with a definite, unvarying value that does not in itself depend on what I know. When I quote confidence limits, I must believe that the true mean either does lie within those limits with certainty (i.e., a probability of 100 percent) or it does not (i.e., a probability of zero)—the 95 percent does not attach to either. Nor does it mean that 95 percent of future sample estimates will lie within these limits. Of course, I do not certainly know which state is true. The value 95 percent is irrelevant except as a statement of *belief*. Now what does that statement mean and what are its warrants?

Let me first try to grapple with the nature of uncertainty.

One extreme view is that since the true mean can never be exactly known with certainty from a finite sample, it is meaningless to suppose that it exists: that the only realities are our own rational and well-founded beliefs; and that there is no point in trying to transcend them.

Another view is that we should distinguish two kinds of probabilities corresponding to two kinds of uncertainty. We may be uncertain either because the answer is in principle unknowable (*objective indeterminacy*) or because it is in principle knowable but is in fact unknown (*subjective uncertainty* or, in Samuel Johnston's blunter terms, "pure ignorance").

Example 5.9. In our genetics clinic we may be consulted by a woman who is a known carrier of hemophilia. She wants to know the risk to her next child and (leaving aside fanciful elaborations and oddities—new mutations and whatnot) we quote a figure of about one in four, since each son is at 50 percent risk, each daughter is at a negligible risk, and the sex ratio is roughly 1:1. Now this figure is equally applicable in two quite different circumstances. It applies if the woman is not pregnant, in which case the issue is not yet, even in principle, decided. But it also applies if she is, say, one month pregnant, too early for either the sex or the phenotype of the fetus to be determined by amniocentesis; but in principle the genotype of the fetus is already determined. In some ways these two expressions of uncertainty are equivalent: for instance, from an actuarial standpoint or as an issue of personal decisions. But in other ways they are quite different. For instance, so long as the woman does not become pregnant, the objective probability statement does not change. But the subjective probability statement will change as the sex of the child gets to be known, either to 0 percent if the fetus is female or to 50 percent if male. If a method of intrauterine diagnosis of hemophilia were available and performed on her, the probability would in some pregnancies rise higher still, perhaps (depending on the reliability of the test) to certainty. In contrast, our current belief is that the sex and genotype of the fetus are irrevocably determined at conception; if so, the (true but unknown) probability in any particular established pregnancy is unchanging at either 0 percent or 100 percent.

Relationship of Confidence Limits to Probability

In some ways a confidence statement is somewhat similar to a subjective probability, in that it would not arise if the observer knew all the facts that are, in principle, available; but it differs, in being a statement about a quantity (the value of a parameter), not about a state (genotype). Until we decide on a definite population to study, there are, perhaps, many possible values that the particular mean level of uric acid may assume. We may even be able to say that 95 percent of the true means for all the various populations lie between 3 and 5, so that the chance of picking one of those that does is 0.95. That is an ordinary objective probability statement. But once the subpopulation has been selected, there is, in principle at least, one perfectly definite answer, whether we know it or not. Confidence limits, then, are not statements about general truth, but represent our beliefs about one particular truth. Like today's newspaper, they have no lasting meaning at all unless we are up against some impenetrable barrier that deprives us permanently of all further information. (This might be true, say, of historical or archeological fact.) Even then it is a statement, not about any property of the unknown, but about the knowledge and ignorance that we have about it from a definable sample of data.

Here two cautions are to the point.

Many probabilists will not like my use of the term *subjective probability,* which they employ in a rather different sense. They use it as a statement of implication. A subjective probability to them corresponds to the odds that a rational, well-informed man would give or take on some particular outcome. That is, their statement appears primarily to deal, not with what is true, but with how the scientist would respond to the data (and by implication what he would empirically believe). Since knowledge changes, the subjective probabilist would not be in the least shocked that probabilities should change. But the objective probabilist expects probabilities to settle down to some definite value. The geneticist, for instance, believes that the probabilistic structure is a permanent feature of Mendelian genetics, not merely a temporary gap in our knowledge. In a famous essay, R. A. Fisher (33) cast some doubt on the authenticity of Mendel's original published data: that his data fitted his model too closely; that one would have expected a greater discrepancy to have occurred from chance variation. This criticism, warranted or not, is certainly of a novel form that would have sounded strange to the Victorian determinist. In particular, it suggests that the chance variation is not merely an imperfection in the data, but a very hallmark of its authenticity.

However, there is a second divergence of views that may be mentioned. To me, a subjective probability statement is not in the least personal. Two competent genetic counselors, presented with the same data, and the same genetic principles, will arrive at the same assessment of risk for a particular pregnant woman. But some subjectivists think it appropriate for the probabilist to include in the analysis all manner of elusive and informal insights. I would call the latter type of statement a *personal probability*. I have no doubt that geniuses work in such a personal fashion. So do fools. The utility of a personal probability statement cannot be weighed without a method of assessing the competence of the person concerned. I am afraid that the abuses of personal probabilities so far outweigh the advantages that while they may serve as a personal guide, there is little place for expressing them in scientific communications. But at the least, one should be able to distinguish among the more, and the less, personalistic components of any probability statement. By this token, *a confidence statement is subjective but not personal.*

Pragmatic Interpretation of Confidence Limits

How, then, are we to interpret a confidence statement? The least controversial statement is in terms of policy and prediction. If a statistician or a group of statisticians have the policy that in analyzing data of a certain type, they will go through a standard procedure to obtain 95 percent confidence limits and, having done so, say that the true value (mean, or whatever is at issue) lies within those limits, then they will be right 95 percent of the time. However, they will not know at the time, if ever, which 95 percent of their decisions are correct.

PROBLEMS

5.1. It is horrendously difficult (and, at the present time, unfeasible) to determine the exact number of people living in the world at any particular instant in time. Does that mean that, even in principle, there is no true answer? Discuss this problem and consider the implications of the possible solutions.

5.2. A circular photographic plate 10 cm in radius is put out into the open. On it is marked off a square with 10 cm sides. If all parts are equally likely to be hit by a cosmic ray, the probability that the first cosmic ray that hits the plate is inside the square is $1/\pi$. As is well known, π cannot be expressed as the ratio of two whole numbers, and (of course) neither can its reciprocal. But the estimate of the proportion based on any finite sample will consist of the ratio of two whole numbers, and thus cannot equal the true probability. Discuss the implications of this example.

5.3. The estimate of the proportion of deaths in a particular type of operation is 10 percent, and the standard deviation is 7 percent. A surgeon believes that because the size of his sample is large, he may suppose the estimate is approximately normal (Gaussian), and he finds the approximate 95 percent confidence limits on the risk of mortality by taking two standard deviations on either side of the mean. Follow his method out, and comment on the results.

5.4. The investigator proposes to estimate the mean of a distribution from a sample of n values, by adding the values and dividing by various quantities: by n, by $(n - 1)$, and by $2n$. Which of these estimators is (a) unbiased; (b) consistent?

5.5. There has been a well-publicized instance (see, for instance, H. Wainer, "Pyramid power: Searching for an error in test scoring with 830,000 helpers," *American Statistician* 37:87–91, 1983) of a multiple-choice question set in a national examination in which because of a subtlety overlooked by the examiners, the official "correct" answer was absolutely wrong. (By absolutely wrong, I mean that precisely because the correct answer is known exactly, its wrongness cannot be disputed). Now there is no redress in examination for this wrong, because the system of examination does not tolerate arguments. In biology many, perhaps most, answers are not, and cannot be, absolutely right. Consider seriously what the implications of multiple-choice questions are for (a) the examination of competence, (b) the resolution of differences between the candidate and the examiner as to what is true, and (c) redress for errors or (more commonly) misjudgments on the part of the examiner.

6 | Conjecture

We have seen that coherent science, like coherent diagnosis, involves the systematic collection and interpretation of pertinent facts. However, this recipe leaves unsolved the question of which interpretations are pertinent and why. A comprehensive answer would not be at all easy to find. In this chapter we shall address one major formal component of it: conjecture, or surmise. In effect, conjecture consists of making a tentative statement; analyzing its consequences and the predictions one would draw from it; and testing to see whether the predictions are fulfilled empirically.

Conjecture is a major activity with diverse forms. The topic is treated usually in a rather piecemeal fashion, dealt with by various kinds of experts in isolation from each other. By taking a broader approach, I shall try to avoid some of the confusions that commonly result from incongruous application of the various methods.

THREE TYPES OF CONJECTURES

We can, at least roughly, divide scientific conjecture into three major groups: formal, structural, and empirical.

Formal Conjecture

This type is the study of the mathematical consequences of a surmise. As such, it deals with abstract *quantities* and *proportions* divorced from all immediate biological components. The most familiar form (which we shall deal with in some detail later) is what is known in Statistics as hypothesis testing. Typically, the drive of the scientist using this method is *refutation* of a hypothesis. Most often he puts up a conjecture (the *null hypothesis*), not with any conviction that it is true, but as a logical device for proving its contrary.* It is like Euclid's method of reduction to the absurd: proving that something must be true by showing that any contrary belief leads to a contradiction, or, in Euclid's case, an impossibility. As we shall see, the chief criterion of proof in such instances is the *significance level*. In general, the hypothesis that is abandoned is perfectly explicit; that which is accepted by default may sometimes be clearly stated but is usually rather vague. If the null hypothesis is that the mean age of a population is sixty, it takes little imagination to devise an alternative hypothesis—that it is greater than sixty; or less than sixty; or that it is either less than or greater than sixty. This method of conjecture is widely used in biological science; it is perhaps insufficiently realized that *such hypotheses are always about quantity.*

Example 6.1. To speak of using this approach to test the null hypothesis that "alcohol does not cause cirrhosis" is not correct. Statistical theory is not concerned with the biochemistry of what one drinks or how cirrhosis is to be observed. Before one can begin the statistical analysis, these scientific ideas must be converted into statistical (quantitative) attributes and numbers. For instance, we might make the null hypothesis "The proportion of people drinking more than 100 ml of alcohol each day who get cirrhosis is no greater than that in those drinking less."

There are other, less familiar, types of formal conjecture (in theoretical physics and applied mathematics, for instance) that are beyond the scope of this book.

Structural Conjectures

These statements are overwhelmingly concerned with surmises about *how the authentic components of a system work.* The statements consist mainly of what are called *models.* Some major biological fields concerned with modeling are genetics, physiology, and ecology (notably the theory of epidemics). In each case, there is a more or less abstract idea of what is happening, abstract in the sense that much of the detail may be ignored and the behavior of certain significant structures alone treated. Further discussion of modeling will be postponed to chapter 11. But a few examples here may help.

Example 6.2. The surmise "The Marfan syndrome is an autosomal dominant disorder" amounts to a statement of two ideas: that the disturbance occurs at one (genetic) locus and that it is

---

*It resembles the oblique method of the borrower ("I don't suppose you could lend me fifty dollars?")—a form used because he realizes that his supposition may be correct, but hopes that it is not.

clinically detectable in the heterozygous state. One, but only one, way of testing that surmise is that certain patterns of segregation are to be expected among the progeny: half to be affected if one parent is heterozygous, three-quarters if both are, and unity if at least one parent is homozygous. In addressing this problem statistically, we have converted a statement about a quality (the Marfan syndrome) to a quantitative statement about segregation ratios in progeny. But this formulation tells us only part of the story.

• *That the predictions are fulfilled does not prove the surmise true.*

Example 6.3. Lilienfeld (34), for instance, found that the empirical facts agree with the predictions of the hypothesis that physicians are the homozygotes for a recessive gene. But nobody, least of all Lilienfeld, believes that this hypothesis is true. He devised the example precisely as an illustration of the dangers of substituting mindless formalism for science.

Conversely, the actual segregation ratios may differ from those predicted by a hypothesis that may very well be true.

Example 6.4. In the disorder incontinentia pigmenti (14), which is arguably an X-linked dominant trait, we would surmise that half the sons and half the daughters of a carrier woman would be affected. In fact, none of the sons are affected, but the total daughters outnumber the sons by 2 to 1. Hemizygous (male) fetuses may be inviable and spontaneously aborted so early in pregnancy as not to be included in our sample. Then the proportion of affected children born to carrier mothers would be, not ½, but ⅓.

However, insofar as scientists, being human, may be allowed to have aspirations, *the preferred outcome from testing structural conjectures will be the exact opposite of that for formal conjectures.* The scientist in this instance hopes that his conjecture is correct and the hypothesis will not be rejected, but will survive searching tests. Now it has been sagely remarked that if the main aim is to preserve a hypothesis, the best plan is not to collect any data at all! To avoid this absurdity, we must change the criterion of success. That used by the scientist engaged in modeling is not the *significance level* (which we shall discuss under Neyman-Pearson Hypothesis Testing), but *power,* or (in more general terms) *falsifiability.* If the conjecture is false, what opportunity has there been to show it false? If no data have been collected, the answer will be none, and the conjecture will have no evidential standing. Conversely, a model that has withstood extreme and exacting tests is on very solid ground. Note, finally, that in contrast with tests of formal conjectures, in this procedure the conjecture being tested is both highly precise and of an essential type; any alternative hypothesis may be so indefinite that one may be unable to formulate it. When a geneticist tests whether the Marfan syndrome is an autosomal dominant disorder, it is not at all clear what he would believe instead should the surmise prove untenable. On the other hand, he can make the trivial surmise about the test criterion that "The segregation ratio assumes some other value." This alternative would command much less respect because it is not at all clear what biological meaning it has.

Example 6.5. The epidemic theorist may argue that the spread of an epidemic may be represented in certain elemental ideas: the carriers, the immune, and the susceptible; infectivity of the organism; the incubation period; the incapacitation and the mortality rates due to the disease; the impact of prevention and treatment. The model will be more elaborate than in example 6.2; but it will also differ in another major respect. In the Marfan syndrome, the segregation ratios (which were the subject of the statistical test) come directly from the logical structure of the model: they are *constitutive parameters*. In the general class of dominant Mendelian traits, the segregation ratios that we surmise are due to the genetic theory about how many genes there are at a locus and how they behave at meiosis. They are the same arguments whatever the trait, and do not belong to the particular disease concerned. By contrast, the epidemic theory tells us nothing about how infectious measles should be or what the incubation period of leprosy should be. These *empirical parameters* will have to be found from experience, often from the data that will be used to test the conjecture. The test then consists of asking "Can we find values of the parameter that will make the model fit best and yet accord with the data?" As one might imagine, the more structures (especially empirical structures) in the model, the more flexible it is, until it would take a vast body of data to give any real power. The wise biologist will at this stage realize that the scientific standing of the model can be rescued only by obtaining intermediate data and not merely by using some global statistic like the total size or duration of the epidemic, which could doubtless be explained by dozens of more or less equally plausible conjectures.

Empirical or Black-box Conjectures
There remain a large group of surmises that are neither primarily quantitative nor logically structured. They deal with relationships at a crassly biological level, such as cannot be cast in elegant abstractions. If they sit long in the sun, fair-skinned people get sunburnt. This relationship might never have been tested scien-

tifically; nor does it need to be—and while we now have quite sophisticated models of the action of ultraviolet light on cells and how the damage it does is repaired, they were not necessary to discover the fact of sunburn, nor have they had to look to quantitative projections for support. A large part of the difficulty of devising a formal study of the subject might be to find a satisfactory measure of exposure and response.

The sophisticated are apt to condescend towards this kind of conjecture; yet it enjoys a number of distinctions not shared by the others. It has a long and successful, even a penetrating, history, as readers of John Stuart Mill would recognize. It is the main, almost the only, source of inspiration for the other kinds of conjecture. Models of genetics started with Mendel conducting experimental studies that involved growing pea plants. Snow had worked out a large part of the logic of epidemics without appealing to a single differential equation. It is sobering to find how often the sophisticated are the late arrivals at what is already a going scientific concern.* Finally, empirical surmise is the ultimate proving ground of the scientific authenticity of either formal or structured conjecture. It is only the outcome of future empirical conjecture that indicates the soundness of the sophisticated model.

Each of these three fields of conjecture has its typical expert. The formal conjecture, because of its abstractness and generality, and because the heart of the problem is almost always random variation, is mostly a matter for the statistician. The structured conjecture, once it gets beyond the most elementary forms, is the domain of the *bio*mathematician, often of the probabilist. Chapter 11 will deal with biomathematical modeling. The empirical conjecture is most typically the concern of the empirical scientist. It is the most elusive area of the three, and to be successfully done, it calls for perceptiveness bordering on genius.

HYPOTHESIS TESTING

It is perhaps not sufficiently realized that there are many ways, even many statistical ways, in which a hypothesis may be tested. The three major methods are those of Bayes, of Fisher, and of Neyman and Pearson. Of the three, the middle one is the most

---

*But there is another side to that question as I shall try to illustrate later under "Prophetic Theories" in chapter 9.

widely used informally; but it is to the other two that I would direct most attention, because they are the most explicitly defined, and their properties are clearest.

In order to pinpoint the issues, it helps to recognize that in evaluating a hypothesis, two questions are involved.

Aptness: How well does the hypothesis explain the available evidence?

Plausibility: How true does it ring?

Example 6.6. Suppose that one morning I find a flat tire on my car. Four of the many possible hypotheses I might put forward are:

1. That the tire may have picked up a nail at the building site nearby.
2. That the puncture is the work of an international conspiracy to make me late for work.
3. That I recall having driven over a black cat on my way home the previous night.
4. That the tire may have been licked by a polar bear looking for honey.

Numbers 1 and 2, if sound, would explain the puncture aptly, whereas the other two would not. Numbers 1 and 3 refer to plausible events; the others do not. The first is the only hypothesis that is apt (nails do cause punctures) and plausible (nails are commonly found at building sites). The fourth is neither plausible (there are few, if any, polar bears at liberty in Baltimore) nor apt (a bear would not puncture a tire by licking it).

Now by the criteria we have previously stated, example 6.6 cannot at once be converted into a test of hypothesis, because it is not cast in terms of quantities and probabilities. But let us keep the image in mind in what follows.

The equivalent to the aptness of a *formal* hypothesis is a conditional statement about the probability of the outcome observed having occurred if the hypothesis is true (and not arguing about the latter assumption). If two parents are carriers of oroticaciduria (which is a rare disease) the probability that two or less of their seven children will be affected is 29/128. (The actual calculations do not matter here.) Note that this *conditional probability* would be the same whatever the frequency of the recessive gene concerned. For instance, if both parents are carriers for the O gene at the ABO blood-group locus (a very common gene), the probability of two or less children being homozygous for blood group O is still 29/128. The point is that the conditional nature of the probability statement means that, however few, or however many, couples we have been able to find, both of whom are carriers of the gene, the probability of any one child *of such a couple* being affected is still one-quarter. So much for aptness. We might say that in example 6.6 the "nail" and the "conspiracy" hypotheses may account about equally well for my flat tire. In the same way, if a child has a dominant trait, present in neither parent, it is equally well explained *if* (for instance) new mutation or nonpaternity has occurred. That is not to say that these two events are equally likely to occur.

But of course, aptness is not enough. The scientist will want to consider plausibility; and in the statistical context, this feature is represented as the *prior probability*. If I lodge a complaint against the Ruritanian embassy for willfully damaging my car, the level-headed and fair-minded policemen may reply that although my hypothesis accounts for the flat tire, it is exceedingly unlikely that that friendly power deliberately punctured my tire for no very clear advantage to themselves. The psychiatric hospitals are full of paranoid patients who have a good enough sense of aptness but no sense of plausibility. The statistician cannot formally handle plausibility except as the prior probability. With these thoughts in mind, let us proceed with the testing of a hypothesis.

First, there must always be at least one possible alternative to the hypothesis put forward; and since, as we have noted, the object of enquiry is always a quantity, finding an alternative is not usually a problem. However apt, the alternative must usually have some empirical plausibility. I cannot imagine a scientist setting out to test the hypothesis "Everybody dies once," simply because there exists a formal alternative, "Everybody dies twice." Once it is conceded that there are at least two hypotheses to be considered, we may take two courses: treat them symmetrically or not.

What do we mean by this distinction?

Bayesian Hypothesis Testing

In the Bayesian method* we treat them symmetrically. That method does not require us to suppose that they are equally plausible; but it involves two rules (which, in fact, say the same thing).

1. There is no *onus* of proof. Neither hypothesis is "in possession." To take a familiar example, in Anglo-Saxon law a person is presumed innocent until proved otherwise. If the prosecu-

---

*This method is so called because it stems from a famous theorem on probability algebra discovered by Thomas Bayes in the eighteenth century.

tion makes an inadequate case, the person will *by default* be declared not guilty, even if there is no attempt by the defense to show the person innocent. The onus of the proof in that case lies on the prosecution.

2. The choice between (or among) the hypotheses, of which one at most can be true, is made on their relative merits. What are these merits? They are the counterparts of aptness and plausibility. Broadly, they are the pieces of evidence available in support of them. The evidence is of two main kinds. The least controversial is the interpretation of certain agreed facts in the light of the hypothesis. Suppose that we treat a randomly selected group of ten patients suffering from a disease, usually fatal, with a new treatment, and all recover, whereas none of a random group of ten controls treated with a placebo does. Then these outcomes are readily explained by the first hypothesis: that the new treatment is effective; it is explained, less readily, by the second hypothesis: that the diagnosis in every patient in the treated group happens to have been mistaken, or that by chance the patients randomly put in the treated group turned out to be the mildest, or at least the luckiest, cases. There would be a general agreement among experts as to how the evidence from the relative plausibilities at this latter level are to be assessed. One can state precisely the probability that, with proper methods of randomization, the ten best cases will happen to fall in the treated group and the ten worst in the control group.

    The second component of merit is at least as important, but often both elusive and controversial. It is the evidence that is at hand before the experimental data are collected at all.

Example 6.7. We may know from massive evidence that penicillin does not cure tuberculosis. The evidence comes from various studies, partly in vitro, partly clinical, partly theoretical. Yet an investigator, using methods that are beyond reproach and working under the most stringent scrutiny, may find that his ten cases treated with penicillin recover and the ten controls all die. Now to be sure, this is an unlikely outcome: about one chance in a million if penicillin has no effect. But *unlikely outcomes do happen, even if they are unlikely.* If they could not happen, we would not call them unlikely; we would call them impossible. It may seem very strange that this particular extreme outcome has occurred if penicillin really is inert in this disease; but we could only conclude from it that penicillin is effective by supposing that the current view founded on all the other controlled trials and the other scientific evidence is wrong, which is even more unlikely.

Just as the physician may be concerned with both general scientific truths and individual diagnoses, so may he also deal with hypotheses about both generalities and particular patients. It is in the latter class that the prior probability is most readily accepted.

Example 6.8. An area of quantitative prognosis that is now well entrenched is rational genetic counseling. To make predictions about the risks that future children will be affected by a Mendelian trait, it suffices to know the genotypes of the persons considering having children. However, the phenotype is often uncertain, because carriers are indistinguishable from noncarriers. So we set up rival hypotheses about the parental genotypes, and in this class of problem we can often assign exact prior probabilities to them. Alice is known to be a carrier of the gene for the X-linked disorder hemophilia (for instance, because her father was affected by it); then Betty (her daughter) has a probability of 1/2 of inheriting the gene. Betty's daughter, Celia (an only child), has thus a prior probability of 1 in 4 of being a carrier and 3 in 4 of not being a carrier. These quantities are the prior probabilities in the sense that we can calculate them even from knowing Celia's relationship to the obligatory carrier, Alice, and without using any other information. The 3 chances in 4 that Celia is not a carrier are made up from 2 chances in 4 (or 1 chance in 2) that Betty does not inherit the gene from her mother and therefore cannot transmit it, and 1 chance in 4 that Betty does inherit it but does not transmit it to Celia. Suppose that Celia is the prospective parent on behalf of whom advice is being sought. Then for practical purposes we may reassure her *if she is not a carrier;* but we would tell her that each of her sons will be at risk *if she is a carrier.* If she has already had two sons, both normal, we may argue that she has had two opportunities to show she is a carrier if she is one; and since both sons are normal, we have a certain amount of evidence against the idea that she is a carrier. Then the prognosis for her next son will be somewhat more optimistic. If one or both sons are affected, we are assured she is a carrier. The details may be found in various books on genetic counseling (35–37).

Example 6.9. Suppose that geneticists are trying to determine on which chromosome a particular gene is carried. In the main, they will rely on empirical evidence of a technical character (e.g., linkage analysis, cell hybridization, the phenotypic effects of deletions, and translocations). But they may also color the analysis by prior probabilities. If it is known or believed (e.g., from looking at cells) that there are ten times as many genes in chromosome 1 as there are in chromosome 21, then they may reasonably start out with the probability that a gene is ten times as likely to be on the former as on the latter. To *offset* this prior slant, the geneticist will need empirical evidence that will make chromosome 21 ten times the more likely one. At that stage the betting would be even; and further evidence will tilt the scales appropriately.

Now let us consider these two last examples. It is assumed that in both cases there is, in principle, an answer that is a definite fact. Celia either is or is not a carrier; the gene either is or is not on chromosome 21. Where then does probability come into it? Well it is clear that these statements are not at all of the same kind as the statement that the probability that Alice's *next* son being affected is 1/2. The statement about the site of a gene is cast as a probabilistic one because of *ignorance of an actual state;* and with further knowledge it may be replaced by certainty. But the genotype of a future son, as yet unconceived, is not yet established because the son does not even exist; and (in my view of the world at least) it is, in the nature of things, impossible to predict with certainty what his genotype will prove to be.* One probability reflects the uncertainty of current knowledge, and since the indeterminacy is subjective, it seems appropriate to call it a subjective probability. The genotype of a future son is uncertain because of the nature of things; and it may be called an objective probability.† This argument should by now be rather familiar. It is very much the statement made about confidence limits in chapter 6, except that it is dealing with states, not values.

Examples 6.8. and 6.9 differ from each other in a fundamental way. The former is a purely individual statement, and because of its private character, it is of little scientific interest; it is incurably particular, and while it has claims to be a scientifically accredited fact, it lacks the august status of a scientific truth. In contrast, the habitual location of a genetic locus in human genomes purports to be a general property of the species, and by and large it will be based on, and applicable to, an entire group. For the most part, it is easier to devise plausible prior probabilities for particular hypoth-

---

*There are those who would argue that, if we knew enough about the exact factors in the fertilization, we could say with certainty which sperm would fertilize which ovum and hence what the genotype of the progeny would be. I cannot imagine how this claim could be proved; and even if it could, it would be of no practical use to the genetic counselor.

†The reader is again warned that not all probabilists use the terms *objective probability* and *subjective probability* in these senses.

eses than for general; and the reason is, I think, that a general scientific truth is much less likely to deal with particular quantities or particular states. Any prior probabilities that there are tend to come from experience. We would be hard-pressed to make a probability statement about how many thoracic vertebrae there ought to be, if we had not counted them in many people. It is not easy to devise prior probability statements about whether a treatment will be beneficial in multiple sclerosis, even if the reasonable physician may feel that particular claims are implausible. A diet of stewed camels' kidneys may work; but it would take a great deal of empirical evidence to convince us that it does, because it does not sound convincing. On the other hand, stranger cures have been discovered, and a rational explanation has subsequently been found. What then is the clinician to do when faced by such claims in which the prior probabilities are difficult to state with even rough precision? Here much controversy starts. Some statisticians would say that even if one can make only the crudest of prior statements about the probabilities that various competing hypotheses are true, one should still make use of them and carry through the argument in the same fashion as in the problem in genetic counseling.

Neyman-Pearson Hypothesis Testing

The most widely used solution, however, involves abandoning some of the original goals. In the procedure of Neyman and Pearson we no longer try to make probability statements about what is, and what is not, true. Nor do we try to conserve symmetry in the way we treat competing hypotheses. Instead, our formal analysis is confined to the empirical data, and we judge the outcome informally, in the light of our background knowledge and our preconceptions.

Let us examine the foregoing argument a little more carefully. In example 6.8 we ask two formal questions.

1. What probabilities would we quote that the daughter of a carrier of hemophilia is (*a*) a carrier and (*b*) not a carrier, before we know anything at all about the daughter or her children? The answers may be regarded as background information before we know the particulars of the case, and we have therefore called them *prior probabilities*.
2. What is the probability that both her sons are normal, (*a*) *if she is a carrier*, and (*b*) *if she is not a carrier*? Both the latter probabilities are based on certain logical conditions (in italics) and are appropriately called *conditional probabilities*. In theory, the phe-

notype of the prospective parent herself gives us some information; but since the disease is recessive, her phenotype will be much the same whether she is affected or not.

When the answers to corresponding parts of two sets of questions are multiplied together, we get the *joint probabilities,* which show the relative plausibilities of the competing hypotheses; and suitably rescaled, they give their *posterior probabilities.* The latter quantities may be viewed as the best and most up-to-date statements one can make.

In example 6.8 the prior probability (fig. 6.1A) that Celia is not a carrier is 3/4. If she is a carrier, the probability (fig. 6.1B) of having two normal sons (each being independently at a risk of 1/2) is 1/4. The other three, equally probable, outcomes (i.e., that only the first son is normal, that only the second is, and that neither is) do not square with the data (that both sons are, in fact, normal). But if she is not a carrier, it is virtually certain that her sons will be normal.

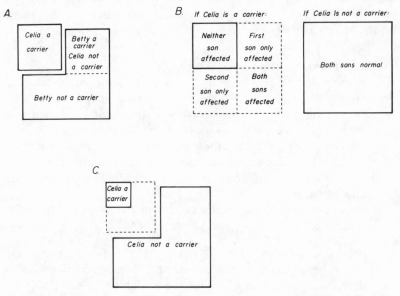

Figure 6.1. A problem in genetic counseling. *A:* The *prior probabilities* for Celia's two possible phenotypes (carrier and noncarrier), and their origins. *B:* The *conditional probabilities* for the various combinations of the sons' phenotypes according to the genotype of Celia. (New mutation is ignored.) The dashed lines enclose outcomes contrary to the facts and therefore not admissible. *C:* The products of *A* and *B*, rescaled to give a unit area. The two figures enclosed in continuous lines represent the *posterior probabilities.*

Table 6.1. A Problem in Genetic Counseling Solved by the Neyman-Pearson Method

Raw Data	Distribution	
Sons affected (outcome)	Number affected (random variable)	Probability of outcome and of value of random variable
Neither	0	0.25
First or second	1	0.5
Both	2	0.25

The joint probability for the carrier hypothesis (fig. 6.1C) is thus (1/4)(1/4) = 1/16; and that for the noncarrier hypothesis is (3/4)(1) = 12/16, which is twelve times as large.

If the same problem were dealt with by the Neyman-Pearson method of testing hypotheses, the argument would go as follows. We begin with the null hypothesis: that (the woman being a carrier) the probability of a son being affected is 1/2. Then the possible outcomes for the two sons would give the distribution shown in table 6.1.

Two further steps are necessary to complete the Neyman-Pearson analysis. We must specify an alternate numerical hypothesis: in this case, that (the woman not being a carrier) the risk of any son being affected is zero. Second, we cannot answer with certainty the question of whether or not the mother is a carrier. So if we are ever to take the gamble of saying she is a carrier, we must decide how much risk we are prepared to take of falsely rejecting the null hypothesis if it is true. (Tests that do not accept some such risk are almost always useless tests.) If this risk is set at (say) 5 percent, we speak of "testing the hypothesis at the 5 percent level." It is commonly written "$p = 0.05$." This latter figure, 0.05, which is chosen freely and arbitrarily by the scientist, is commonly called *the level of statistical significance.**

The answer to the analysis is then whether—given the null hypothesis—the chance of the outcome (or something more extreme still) is 5 percent or less, in which case we reject the hypothesis; or failing that, we accept the hypothesis.

Note several points.

*More strictly, this percentage is called *the size* of the test if it is chosen before the data are collected and *the significance level* if it is chosen after the result of the analysis is known.

1. The significance level *is not a direct probability statement about the hypothesis, given the data.* It is a conditional probability statement *about the data, given the hypothesis.* It may not be easy to explain the data, given the hypothesis; but it may be even more difficult to explain it under any other surmise.
2. The verdict does not depend on how much more readily some other hypothesis would explain the data. We do not even start to take that question seriously until we have rejected the null hypothesis.
3. Some investigators choose the risk of falsely rejecting the null hypothesis after the data have been examined. They do this in such a way that they would barely reject the null hypothesis if it were true. For instance, suppose it turns out that if the null hypothesis were true, 4 percent of the possible outcomes would be more extreme than the one observed. Then they argue that if they had picked the size of the test at 4 percent, they would have barely rejected the null hypothesis. This means that the significance level is then a random variable: were they to repeat the experiment, they should almost certainly reach a different significance level. I have a good deal of sympathy with this argument if we are ever to do justice to the weight of the evidence. But it is not the method prescribed by Neyman and Pearson.
4. The only assured property of the method of Neyman-Pearson is that in a test done strictly at the 5 percent level of significance, *when the null hypothesis is true, we shall on average reject it one time in twenty.* If we call such an outcome significant and follow it up by further experiments, then we will start a maximum of one wild-goose chase for every twenty tests of hypotheses. The better focused the science, the more likely we are to be testing null hypotheses that are indeed false, and the less the risk of a wild-goose chase. In what is known colloquially as a fishing expedition,—that is, a study that consists of amassing data and promiscuously searching for clues—nearly all the leads will be false. What is worse, the other kind of geese, those that lay the golden eggs, may be missed by chance if individual studies are few and the power is feeble.
5. The statistical significance level is a statement about *evidence*, not about *effect*. If it is small enough, say $p = 0.001$, we infer that the result is not readily explained as a chance outcome if the null hypothesis is true; and we start to look for an alternative explanation with considerable assurance. But the alternative we find may still be only trivially different from the null.

Example 6.10. Suppose that large doses of vitamin C reduce the average number of colds per winter from 2.80 to 2.79 per person; if the study is large enough, this difference may be highly significant statistically. In time, it may lead to important discoveries. However, the therapeutic impact is trivial. Vitamin C would clearly have something definite to do with the common cold, but very little. (To my mind, this case calls for estimation: finding the *magnitude* of the effect is of much more interest than testing a hypothesis about it.)

If we apply the Neyman-Pearson system of hypothesis testing to our problem in genetic counseling, the most extreme outcome possible under the null hypothesis would be that observed: that no sons are affected. The probability of that outcome, as we have seen, is 25 percent; thus, we would reject the null hypothesis at the 25 percent level. We cannot construct a test at the 5 percent level at all; so by the common arbitrary criterion, we accept the null hypothesis and declare the woman a carrier. This conclusion is anomalous when, as we found above, the outcome from the Bayesian analysis tells us that the odds are 12 to 1 that she is not a carrier.

Is there any redress for this unsatisfactory outcome from the Neyman-Pearson approach? In principle, there are two. First we look at *the power of the test*, that is, the probability of rejecting the null hypothesis if it is false. In example 6.8 we have seen that we can never reject the null hypothesis at the 5 percent level at all; hence, the power is zero. This tells us that it is useless to aspire to that degree of assurance on the conditional probability derived from two sons only. If the issue were a scientific one (and therefore a general or generalizable one), the solution would be to collect more data. However, genetic counseling is not a scientific activity but a clinical one. We cannot get more data (i.e., ask the woman to have more sons) in order to answer her question as to whether she should have more sons. And even if we could, the answer would be perpetually changing and always out of date. For as each son is born, we should be trying to find the risk for the next one, on a steadily increasing body of data.

More generally, to solve any diagnostic problem in an individual patient, it is rarely possible to gain more information about the individual by examining other people. (Occasionally, there is help from examining the relatives or the contacts in inherited or communicable diseases, respectively.) In this respect, diagnosis is more akin to probability algebra than to statistics. One is making statements that are, in a sense, predictive, about an individual person, not making inferences about common properties of a population.

After the event, the predictions are useless. Evidence that 70 percent of patients survive an operation is no comfort to the relatives of the patient who dies during it, and it is lukewarm assurance to the patient who has already survived.

The other, and more dangerous, recourse is common sense. We judge the meaning of a significance level in the light of experience, calling on analogies, hunches, and so forth. I have no doubt that most people would be bored writing out a telephone directory backwards. Although I know of no evidence on the point, I would believe it even if the significance level were only 10 percent. If it were claimed from the same study that there is a higher rate of cancer in those so engaged than in controls copying it forwards, I would be reluctant to believe the claim, even if the significance level were 0.001. Nevertheless, we can easily think of plenty of instances in which ignorance and bigotry masquerading as common sense have been used, and are still being used, to overtrump sound data. Statisticians of the Neyman-Pearson school would argue that at least the informal background of interpretation (bigotry and all), if stuck on after the formal analysis has been completed, is out in the open: one can distinguish hard analysis from opinion; that on the other hand, the Bayesians who canonize their background (including crass prejudice) build it into the first line of the analysis; and how much it contributes to the final answer is not at all easy to see at later stages in the analysis.

Fisherian Hypothesis Testing

From what *probability* means, the outcome is as likely to be in any 5 percent of the sample space as any other, and hence to give the same significance level. Neyman and Pearson prescribe that the 5 percent be chosen so as to maximize the power. Fisher's ideas on hypothesis testing are obscure and are variously interpreted. Like those of Neyman and Pearson, they are based only on data and ignore priors. However, Fisher flatly rejected the idea of power, and it is unclear how he selected his rejection region; in many common problems it lies in the tails of the curve. This informal pattern is often used by scientists who usually ignore power, and most of the time with impunity. But there are problems when it is unclear where the alternative to the null hypothesis lies. It is hard to be sure what the properties of the procedure are.

THE CLINICAL COMPROMISE

It is my view that in medicine we have taken our responsibilities for the background too lightly. The clinical textbooks contain exquisite descriptions of the features of a disease, and the best of them record explicit statements about how frequently each particular pertinent symptom or sign appears in it and in how severe a degree. This information is rather like the conditional probabilities in the Bayesian system. *If* the patient has a lung abscess, the probability that he will have clubbing of the fingers is *c* percent. But as in the scientific case, the clinician making the diagnosis in a particular patient wants to assess, *not* the probability of clubbing, given a lung abscess, but the reverse conditional probability, that of a lung abscess, given that the patient has clubbing. There are few patients who come complaining of a lung abscess and ask the physician to say whether they have clubbing. Most of those who do have some kind of anxiety state and are usually in need of psychiatric help. The usual pattern is the exact converse.

In the same way, to say that patients with untreated Addison's disease almost certainly have low blood pressure is not at all the same as to say that patients with low blood pressure almost certainly have untreated Addison's disease. We can make the logical transition (the nub of clinical diagnosis: the inverting of the order of such conditional probabilities) only by considering and giving due weight to *all* the other possibilities. We seldom see Japanese river fever in East Baltimore; and the evidence for it would have to be almost compelling before a sensible physician would diagnose it.

Example 6.11. Suppose a well-informed, but inexperienced, physician sees a patient with a four-day history of backache, headache, and fever, followed by a vesicular eruption heaviest on the face, palms, and feet—the vesicles of which become umbilicated. His intellectual satisfaction after consulting the appropriate sources is apt to go in two steps. First, the good news: the conditional probability that these features occur in smallpox is very high. Second, the bad news: the prior probability of smallpox (which the experts tell us is now extinct) is zero.

The gaps in rational diagnosis are that we do not know, or pay little attention to, the prevalence of the diseases we diagnose and the chances that they will come our way; and we know little about the frequency and the severity of the findings to which we appeal in diagnosis. The clinician may make much of recurrent headache in a diagnosis; but do we *really* know what the probability is that a person *taken at random from the reference population* has recurrent headache? Or in dealing with a measurement, say the level of lactic dehydrogenase in the serum, I doubt that most hospitals have figures for the distribution of values in a formal, representative sample from the population that they serve.

The Information That the Clinician Needs

The ideal background for interpreting such data is worth some thought. In starting a new diagnostic test, it is wise to do it properly at the outset and so avoid the makeshift that is then imposed for ethical or legal reasons. In the population of interest, we might ideally proceed as follows.

1. A formal, random sample of people is obtained that is both representative and of adequate size.
2. Those suffering from diseases are set aside for the time being.
3. The conditions for which the laboratory proposes to test are studied, and the factors that influence them: age, sex, race, etc. These characteristics may be related to each other. The results furnish the data against which any results in a future patient are to be interpreted.
4. The diseased people in the sample are used to identify the prevalence of the disease to which the test is pertinent, and what the distributions of values are in these disorders.

In reality, what is usually done is to make a collection of observations, often from a poorly defined population. Little attempt is made to define whether they have diseases, and if so, what diseases. For no very clear reason (certainly not a statistical one), it is supposed that 95 percent of the results (the central, or the lowest, or the highest 95 percent, according to taste) must be healthy, and the rest, if not diseased, are at least suspect. This policy means, as before, that inexorably the healths of 5 percent of healthy persons are needlessly called into question, and the more tests that are done, the greater the risk of at least one of them being in the questionable zone.

Anybody who has introduced a new test knows that my prescription is hard to follow and that a less severe practice is much easier. Even the experts on screening rarely try to gather the information that is necessary for precise and efficient use of the data. The clinician adapts to the demands of the system by not using any laboratory test to make life and death decisions unless the results are extreme. How far this course is to be seen as prudence, and how far as makeshift, I am not prepared to say here, although I have my opinions. But there is little doubt that if the information really needed were at hand, one would be able to make use of the preferred Bayesian approach rather than the rather second-rate Neyman-Pearson method.

Costs, Penalties, and Decisions

What is more, an adequate Bayesian approach would allow us to address two other facets of diagnosis, which the sound and compassionate clinician always had in mind, but which defy a purely probabilistic formulation.

First, what are the consequences of errors of diagnosis? If a treatment is relatively harmless and yet lifesaving in a naturally dangerous disease (as vitamin B_{12} is in subacute combined degeneration of the cord or penicillin is in syphilis), then if one cannot altogether escape some errors, it is better to overdiagnose than to underdiagnose. If there is nothing to be gained from early diagnosis in a disease that is untreatable, then the converse is the case.

Second, expense must be considered in all senses: money, worry, pain, embarrassment, incapacitation, burden on the limited load of patients that can be catered for by a special diagnostic device, etc. The spirit of the age is against me, but I cannot see that there is much to be gained from an expensive, disabling, even dangerous procedure that will make no difference to the management of the patient, even if it satisfies the professional curiosity of his doctor.

I have provided a lengthier discussion of these principles of clinical decision theory elsewhere (11).

PROBLEMS

6.1. Identify the objective and subjective probabilistic components in the following arguments.
  a. Tom, who has a headache, does not have multiple sclerosis, because headache is not a feature of multiple sclerosis.
  b. A person who claims to have stayed for ten minutes under water without breathing apparatus must be lying.
  c. The mother of a son with the Lesch-Nyhan syndrome is almost certainly not a carrier, because the carrier state is extremely rare.

6.2. What is the power of a test when the null hypothesis has been rejected at the 5 percent level?

6.3. Chicken pox (varicella) is fatal in less than 1 in 10,000 cases. It is claimed that a child has died of varicella encephalitis. A pathologist rejects this diagnosis at the 1 in 10,000 level of significance. Comments?

6.4. In a study on the effects of drinking American vodka on cirrhosis of the liver, there is a comment added that where

Russian vodka is concerned, the information (of which there is much less) is insufficient to show that there is any lower risk from it. The statement might just as well be cast in the form that there was insufficient evidence that they are at as great a risk. Analyze the possible reasons why each expression should be used.

6.5. Do men have lower thresholds for pain than women?

6.6. Analyze the following claim. "The experienced scientist has nothing to learn from a junior laboratory technician, who in all respects has less training, less experience, and less knowledge." Consider this same statement when "physician" is substituted for "scientist" and "nurse" for "laboratory technician."

6.7. "If they live long enough, all white horses will die of melanoma." (A melanoma is a malignant tumor of pigment cells.) Without appealing to empirical fact, discuss the nature and implications of that statement. Is it verifiable? Falsifiable?

7 | Random and Nonrandom Variation

In this chapter we shall amplify some ideas casually encountered in previous chapters, treating them in a fashion that will pave the way for the ideas we shall develop in the last section of the book. If it is somewhat repetitive in parts, I make no apology; the issues are of great importance in Medicine. For all that, few seem to take on the task of discussing them.

From a highly refined and respected theory comes the notion that in a communication there are two components.

1. *Message,* which is the business end of the process; it is to be reinforced, safeguarded, made accessible.
2. *Noise,* which is merely a nuisance and is to be kept to a minimum.

These basic ideas are not analyzed in what follows. But I appeal to them as a kind of rough metaphor.

The *message* may be intended information, as when some fact or idea is being communicated from one mind to another through a fallible medium such as speech. Much of the clinician's time is taken up trying to understand the patient's vocabulary and sentence structure. Or again, message may be used to denote the significance of the symptoms that the patient tells him, which may be totally unknown to the patient.

Example 7.1. Consider a patient who has had an epileptic fit while standing on the platform of a railroad station. It may be photic epilepsy and then the fact that he was watching a passing train when he had the fit may be highly significant. The physician may have to dig out many such details.

The physician is forever sorting out what he perceives to be *relevant* to *the issue;* and while it may be proper for him to do so, this course implies that the issue can be defined and that the relevant can be recognized. The professional sense of responsibility calls for some tactical concern about both problems, and a strategic commitment to furthering means to make them clearer.

One shallow view is to translate the term *message* into "mean" or "average," and *noise* into "variance" or "scatter." Unfortunately, this narrow translation is fostered by the many successes of the traditional way of dividing up the data used in what is called analysis of variance. It dominates several branches of science (e.g., experimental design, quantitative genetics, numerical taxonomy, regression analysis). The seductive properties of the success and elegance in these fields have reinforced this perception of reality to the point that many scientists, even some practical statisticians, may find it strange to think in other terms. Some, at least, of the hostility that physicians show when attacking statistics may stem from an unarticulated, even an unconscious, rejection of this seduction. In this chapter we shall see how far the rejection is warranted and what might be done to remedy it.

VARIATION

We may take for granted, however trite the thought, that identifying and conveying information must depend on variation of some kind. If there were no features that let one distinguish between one thing and anything else, why there would be neither content nor means of communicating anything. But how that variation is to be characterized is another matter. The fatal error is to confuse variation (which is a fundamental without which empirical knowledge hardly exists) and variance, which we discussed in chapter 4. Variance is merely one kind of statistical descriptor—usually inadequate, often misleading, at times even an embarrassing myth.

The Mean as a Measure

When those using statistics try to think of variation, they commonly start with a set of sample data, add them (giving "the sum"), and add their squares (the "total sum of squares"). They then manipulate these two quantities (and other sums like them) by the kind of maneuvers discussed in the appendix. Through these maneuvers, they hope to throw light on certain statistical questions. They take for granted that these statistical questions are also scientific questions (as they often are). From the total sum of squares is taken a part "accounted for" by the mean. That is, if one redefines each datum, taking the mean of the sample as a new reference point, the new sum of squares (i.e., from the sample mean) will be less than the original sum of squares by an amount called "the sum of squares due to the mean." Or instead of using only one such value as a point of reference, the statistician may have different points of reference for each age group; and the sum of squares of the difference between each value and its reference point will virtually always be a smaller sum still, because "the effect of age" will also have been taken away (fig. 7.1). Of course it may turn out that there has been no significant effect from age, so that age does not account for any more of the variation than the effect of pure chance. Eventually, inspiration flagging, the statistician gives up on the rest of the sum of squares, which is then labeled, formally, *the residual sum of squares* or, conceptually, *the noise*. The whole endeavor has consisted of making as much as possible of the noise into message or (as the statistician sees it) transferring sums of squares from the "error" part into the "parameter" part. In effect, much of what was at first called variance is found on closer examination not really to be variance at all, but systematic effects.

The Variance as a Measure

The whole business, although strictly orthodox and formally beyond reproach, seems to be at times more or less questionable scientifically. One sees it rather more clearly when such techniques are used to compare populations. "Does drug *A* improve high blood pressure?" becomes converted into the question "Is the mean blood pressure in the treated group less than that in the control group?" The mean value may indeed be the point of the point. But it may not. We shall have some other possibilities to consider later. More narrowly, using the mean alone pays no attention to what the most desirable blood pressure would be. If there is nothing more to therapeutics than lowering the blood pressure, then removing some of the blood from the patient (or even, in desperation, de-capitating him!) will do very well. Let us be content to say that the behavior of the mean tells us *something* about the action of the drug, but not necessarily what we most need to know.

Example 7.2. The drug tetraethylammonium bromide may lower the blood pressure in one subgroup of patients with high blood pressure (such as those with kidney disease) and raise it in others (e.g., those with the endocrine disorder pheochromocytoma), as LaDue and his associates showed (38). Taking the average of the responses indiscriminately mixed together, may more or less completely conceal both facts. Even so, one may argue that in such cases

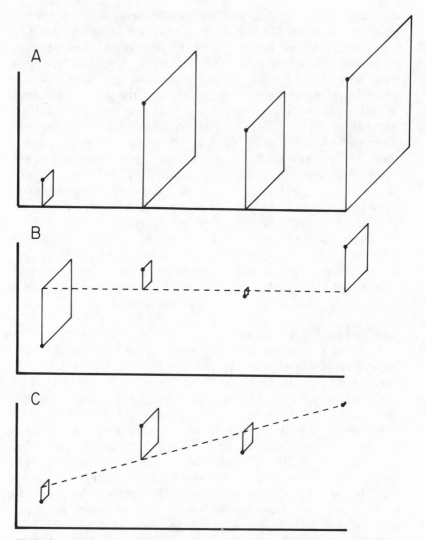

Figure 7.1. Conversion of unidentified variation into systematic effects. In each of the three diagrams, the same four points are plotted. To each is attached a square. *A:* The squares of the original measurements (i.e., the deviation of the values from the baseline of zero). *B:* The squares of the deviations of the data points from the sample mean of all the values (the dashed line). The reduction in the total area of the squares is ascribed to the systematic effect of the mean. *C:* The squares of the deviations from the best-fitting straight line through the points (the dashed line). The further reduction of the sum of the areas from that in *B* represents the (systematic, linear) effect of age.

if, in the analysis, we stratified the patients with sufficient care, we should perceive both effects.

Example 7.3. The drug clonidine is widely used to lower *high* blood pressure. But Robertson and his associates (39) have recently shown that it is an effective way of treating the *low* blood pressure that tends to occur in some patients when standing (postural hypotension). While the mode of action is uncertain, there is reason to believe that the whole story of its effect is not told by the mean alone.

However, in other cases the effect is not on the mean at all.

Example 7.4. Zaimis et al. (40) have shown that it would not be proper to infer that a ganglionic-blocking drug is having no effect on the system that regulates blood pressure simply because in a certain dose it has had no discernible effect on the blood pressure. Indeed, alert physicians noted early that loss of a small quantity of blood (say 250 ml) or prolonged standing or even the skin flushing that occurs on a hot day will produce a profound fall in blood pressure in patients receiving doses of the drug insufficient to produce discernible effect in ordinary circumstances; in contrast, control patients show no such sensitivity. One is tempted to construe this effect as showing that the drug acts on homeostatic processes when it is not yet actively lowering the blood pressure. It is not the *mean* blood pressure that reflects the change due to the drug but the *stability* of the blood pressure.

Example 7.5. The same is true of the mechanisms that regulate the removal of carbon dioxide from the blood. At any time, a certain amount of this gas is retained in the blood to preserve the correct acid-base balance. In certain circumstances the amount retained is excessive, and the patient breathes more deeply to remove it. But sometimes he overbreathes; so he stops breathing altogether to compensate, and overcompensates; then overbreathes again, and so on. This cyclical pattern (Cheyne-Stokes respiration) is characteristic of depressed functioning of the respiratory center, sometimes induced by drugs or by high altitude; it also occurs when the mean transit time between the lungs and the carotid body is prolonged because of a large "central blood volume." It is useless to put forward the argument (as a narrow concern with the mean would prompt) that on average such people have normal blood levels of carbon dioxide and that the variance of their levels is merely noise. It is precisely the variation *within* the individual that contains the significant information, the message about the disordered function. One way of expressing the variation (not, indeed, the best) is to treat the measurements in the several stages of the cycle as if they were random variables and to compute their variance.

Now insofar as one thinks of these correcting devices as being designed to respond adequately to factors that perturb some vital body characteristic, one might suppose that a prompt and energetic response is what is called for, and Cheyne-Stokes respiration is the result of a sluggish response. A sluggish response—and I suppose death is the extreme example—may indeed be harmful. But too brisk a response may lead not only to overcorrection but to a steadily amplifying overcorrection (41); anybody who has seen a patient with an intention tremor, the shake that is aggravated when the patient tries to control fine movement, will understand the process (fig. 7.2). Much of the failure of quantitative genetics to recognize genetic components of measurable characteristics may lie in its preoccupation with heritable variation of values when in many cases it should perhaps be directed to variation of variance (42). And yet the neglect of this topic by geneticists is odd; for it is clear that selection for a particular level of variance has, in princi-

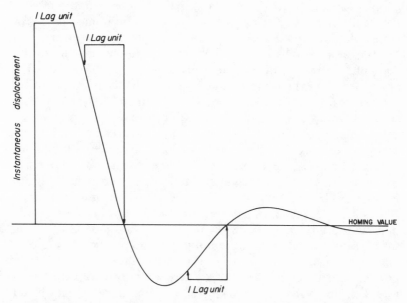

Figure 7.2. Linear homeostasis. At any instant, the adjustment in the system is proportional to what the displacement from the homing value was at a time one lag unit (*L*) earlier. Hence, when it first reaches the homing value (second arrow), it does not stop falling, because it is responding to what the displacement was at the first arrow, one lag unit earlier. The contrary happens at the second crossing. The oscillation will eventually die out.

ple, just as much claim on our attention as selection for a particular mean.

Other Indices

There are a great many other characteristics of a trait that might be the target for selection other than the mean and the variance.

The range is such an instance. Many perturbations have virtually no impact until the extremes are attained, at which point disability follows rapidly. A classic example is the dislocation of a joint; but there are many others that will come to mind. Too much distension of a lung will rupture it; too little will collapse it; but within these critical limits variation has little impact.

Asymmetry ("skewness") may be the main target of selection. Many natural functions (such as walking) depend on balance, and many cyclical functions (such as sleeping, or the sexual cycle in women), to be healthy, depend on a symmetrically wide excursion from one extreme to the other. The psychological composition of a healthy society depends on having a balance of introverts and extroverts, cyclothymes and schizothymes, thinkers and doers, and all the rest.

Modality may be the issue. It may be only the extreme values that are stable states and the intermediate values that are disastrous, so that it is in the *bimodality* (the two-peakedness) of the distribution that the message lies.

Example 7.6. At the onset of labor the safe fetal positions are with the head downwards (vertex presentation) or—rather less safe—upwards (breech presentation): it is the intermediate degrees of rotation (transverse lie) that are dangerous. Likewise, during labor it is best that the occiput rotate either forward or (more rarely) backward. It is the neutral position (deep transverse arrest) that is the dangerous one.

Randomness as Message

It will be evident that in all the foregoing examples we are at least demanding that the message be in the form of a definite quantity. The values may vary randomly, but the true mean itself is a nonrandom constant. The values vary randomly around the true mean, but the variance, the range, the skewness, and so forth, although measurements of random variation, are themselves constants. But to the occult determinists, it may come as a shock to find that at times the message lies, not in any deterministic component, but precisely in randomness of the process. Two examples may suffice.

Example 7.7. The recent discoveries about the origin of antibodies suggests that their specificities are controlled by random piecing together of staple components that are already in stock and available from the genome (43); that when by chance an effective combination of parts occurs, the cells that produce it multiply rapidly. The number of combinations far exceeds the number of types of components. Thus, because of the added virtue of random assemblage, the repertoire of responses exceeds the number of components, a thousandfold or more. It is not the phenotypes that are genetically determined but *the apparatus for randomly generating them.* No doubt the random method is jealously conserved by evolution.

Example 7.8. Another such genetically patterned randomness is seen in the process of Lyonization, the random inactivation of all but one X chromosome in each cell (24). Thus, clones from different lines of cells exhibit random variation that matches what would be predicted from theory. Presumably this is the device for adjusting the chromosomal imbalance that results from incorrect numbers of chromosomes due to accidents in meiosis. The resulting disruption is far less severe than occurs in anomalies of the number of autosomes (i.e., nonsex chromosomes).

A random process may exhibit somewhat confusing behavior in the individual event, but at least one can make precise statements about the corporate behavior of events. We cannot predict how soon the next disintegration from a source of the radionuclide ^{32}P will take place; but we can state the half-life of ^{32}P with high precision. Furthermore, the distribution of the number of counts per unit time follows the so-called Poisson distribution. The physicist uses precisely the distribution of results to check that there is no contaminating source (e.g., electrical interference) in the particle counter. Radioactive decay is a random process but not a chaotic one.

Chaos as Message

But there is an even more unsettling possibility, which I face with some apprehension: that the message may sometimes be chaos. The only respects in which we can characterize chaos are purely negative: that it cannot be described.

To be sure, it is, by definition, impossible to show positively that a process is chaotic, for the obvious reason that chaos has no testable properties. One can always compile a histogram of individual observations; but unless this histogram has some coherence (at the very least that the histograms from several such large studies will tend progressively to resemble each other as the sample sizes increase), there comes a point at which the burden of proof lies on those that believe there is anything there but chaos.

Yet I can think of instances in Medicine that appear to be chaotic: they cannot be described except by pure negatives, and that is precisely how they are recognized. I cite two instances with which every competent physician is familiar. To my knowledge, nobody has even assembled any evidence to suggest that they are anything other than chaotic.

Example 7.9. There is a disordered rhythm of the heart known as *atrial fibrillation,* in which that structure in the atrium that normally sets the rhythm of the heartbeat ceases to function; and the ventricular contractions (which are normally triggered by regular atrial impulses from it) are now triggered in a haphazard fashion by whatever impulses come near. The diagnosis of this disorder is perhaps best made by the electrocardiogram; but it would be a poor physician who could not make a fairly confident diagnosis of it at the bedside. The pattern to watch out for is a complete absence of pattern. The heart rate is often, though by no means always, fast, and it may vary spontaneously and irregularly from minute to minute in the same patient.

Example 7.10. There is a condition known as (Sydenham's or rheumatic) *chorea,* a word incongruously derived from the Greek verb "to dance." It is a usually transient disorder of the nervous system in which from time to time the patient makes rather quick, spontaneous, involuntary movements of what are ordinarily voluntary muscles. It is typically a concomitant of rheumatic fever, which is one of the diagnostic clues. At a casual glance, the movements may be confused with nervous tics; but they differ in that they exhibit no repetitive pattern at all, either in time or in space. Indeed, self-conscious patients acquire great skill in masking them, deftly converting a sudden involuntary action into a smooth movement that may appear to be purposive. Such people may appear to be merely fidgety; and sometimes it may take even the expert observer several minutes of unobtrusive observation to decide whether the person really has the chorea. In theory, the condition could be simulated by a skilled hysteric; but in fact, it is difficult to produce a succession of movements with no regularity whatsoever in the pattern.

In both these examples, the diagnosis rests on the total lack of pattern, even, so far as one can judge, of any probabilistic pattern. Whether a detailed analysis would show that the location, timing, and size of the movements can ultimately be represented as a distribution, I cannot say. But as the clinician sees the condition, it is a formless pattern.

Note a subtle point that arises from the contrast between the last two ideas. It would be a perceptive eye that, simply by looking, could tell randomness from chaos. One of the clues is some underlying sameness in the randomness; and closer inspection may show that it is not random at all.

Example 7.11. A classical example is the famous dance of the harvesting bee. The great naturalist Fabre, despite a lifetime of observation, seems either not to have noted it at all, or to have decided it was of no importance (44). Carefully controlled studies by von Frisch (45) showed that this apparently pointless movement was a means of transferring quite sophisticated information to the other bees about the direction and distance of sources of food.

HIDDEN MESSAGE

So far, we have addressed those types of message that may be discernible by (as it were) tuning in on the correct statistical wavelength. If the message is not evident in the mean, it may lie in some other formal feature amenable to analysis. But it is possible that the meaning may be, not analytically hidden, but evident at a more profound and arbitrary, or conventional, level. Such is the use of the genetic code as a means of transmitting instructions on the assembly of proteins. This deeper probing may also be used as a source of a message that is not in any sense purposeful at all.

Example 7.12. One illustration comes from seeing the genetic message at the level, not of amino acids, but of nucleotides. For, granted that the code is arbitrary, and granted that it is to be expressed in terms of four nucleotides in a triplet code, the translation into nucleotides can tell us, for instance, whether a particular amino acid substitution demands at least one or two or three nucleotide substitutions. What the answer is may give information on the mutation rate at that particular site, depending on how different mutational events may be distinguished (46). For instance, I am indebted to Dr. Kirby Smith for a list of several hemoglobins that, although differing from the usual type in only one amino acid, can only have been produced by two separate nucleotide substitutions (table 7.1).

The Autochthonous

This bizarre word, in wide use among psychiatrists, denotes whatever is "native where it arises"; that is, it is not prompted by

Table 7.1. Minimum Complexity of Mutations in the Beta Chain of Hemoglobin

Type of Hemoglobin	Position	Substitution	Comment
S	6	GAA to GUA	At least one change
C Harlem[a]	6	GAA to GUA	As in sickle
	73	GAA to AAU	At least two changes
None known	—	—	At least three changes

[a]This hemoglobin has mutated at two points.

any outside cause; nor is it generated by a formalized randomizing device. In some ill-understood way, it has meaning, purpose, importance—features that at once distinguish it from the chaotic. Despite its elusiveness, I mention it here for two reasons. First, it may be helpful in rescuing readers from the tyranny of the balance sheet: from the constraining notion that there is anything in the foregoing list that by its very nature guarantees that it is exhaustive and that it ever entitles us to say that something must be chaotic because we have shown that it can neither be caused nor random. In my most committed opinion, that is bad science, very bad logic, and deplorable medicine. Second, there are reasons for believing that there are events of this kind. To be sure, nothing but harm will come from using this notion as an intellectual bolthole, something that we appeal to when we lack the inspiration, courage, purpose, or means to pursue sound scientific enquiry. On the other hand, a morbid fear of saying "I do not know" or "I do not understand" has led, among scientists, to the most preposterous cramming of round pegs into square holes. Some of the shallower surmisal has tried to "explain away" art, freedom, scientific discovery and other inspirations, creativity, sense of value, and much more.

Despite the discursive nature of this book, it is not all about everything. Nor do I for a moment suppose myself competent to deal with the autochthonous, with that which has meaning from within. But, however superficially, I realize that at least some of the variation exhibited by patients is not to be crassly thrust aside as meaningless because it cannot be wholly encompassed by the paradigms of science that we know of so far. I do not believe that good clinicians are made on these terms.

One could cite various devices by which one mechanism may cover the tracks of another in such a way as to conceal both. It is not

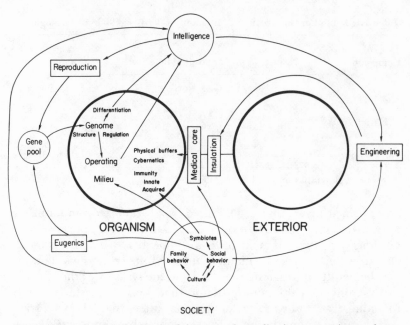

Figure 7.3. A simplified schema of the correcting, adjusting, protecting, and concealing mechanisms in a sophisticated, reflective, and social animal. (Reproduced from the *American Journal of Medical Genetics* [47], by kind permission of the editor.)

surprising that such mutual concealment should occur; for a major trend in evolution is to interpose buffers between the vital parts of the organism and the environment (see fig. 7.3). As examples of the mechanisms involved, one thinks of physical, immune, and homeostatic barriers; social and behavioral patterns; intelligence and its products, such as engineering (47). To some extent, then, these selfsame mechanisms will tend to render the organism inaccessible to the less subtle probing devices. For the common way to study one component of a system is to perturb that part of it. But we may be frustrated in the attempt by these very compensating devices, which may be overcome only by means that may, by their artificiality and disruptiveness, call into question the validity of any conclusion.

Example 7.13. Suppose that we argue that the venous return influences the cardiac output and hence the blood pressure. The question is, perhaps, how big the effect is. Well, one simple test is to see the effect of standing (which, by gravity, reduces the venous return). However, this effect is largely masked by reflex constriction of the arterioles. Exquisite studies have been done on the effect of posture after vasoconstriction has been blocked phar-

macologically i.e., by drugs; but their pertinence to normal physiology is in some question, because other aspects of the car-
diovascular system are affected at the same time by those drugs.

It is certainly no secret that elucidating normal physiology may
call for considerable subtlety and finesse and that the magnitude of
the problem is at its height in the most elaborately buffered physiological system of all, the brain. As to the mind, the insulation is so
much more subtle as to leave the warrant for psychiatry in permanent jeopardy. For the psychiatric endeavor amounts to one mind
trying to grasp, judge, manipulate, and correct another mind. It is
a relationship between peers or almost peers; and it is not at all
obvious that the undertaking is warrantable in the same terms as a
mechanic may have the warrant to fix a radio set. If the psychiatrist
were denied his own insight, I do not see how one psychiatrist
could treat another, for the gauge is not, of its nature, any more
refined than what is being gauged.

THE TOOLS OF INTERPRETATION

Granted that there is message and granted that it may be difficult to locate and identify, how are we to give it scientific standing?
The naive answers to that question are that truth is manifest, that
we know message when we see it; and that if you have to ask the
question, then the quality of the data is not good enough. This kind
of answer is common among those immersed in nineteenth century
macrophysics who have had little to do either with modern biology
or with particle physics. Certainly in biology there are endless opportunities for reading false patterns into data, and for missing
patterns through being distracted by the irrelevant.

What then are we to do? The answer that has come to be given in
biostatistics is that one shapes up some index that contains whatever evidence there is in favor of a hypothesis and sees how far any
discrepancies between the data and the hypothesis can be explained away by the operation of pure chance (see chapter 6). The
onus of proof rests on those that believe that the hypothesis is
inadequate. This criterion involves us in certain issues that are
neither obvious nor trivial. What is the relationship between the
surmise and the data? What, in this context, do we mean by pure
chance? What is the relationship between the hypothesis and the
design? These three questions are intimately related. Let us try to
deal with them in order.

Surmise and Data

It is a common view of science, to which I subscribe but which I
am hard put to defend, that surmise before the fact is more power-

ful than that after the fact. Parts of this arrangement are easy to see. A responsible surmise before the fact (which then has to face the tribunal of empirical testing) must be squarely based on prior data and the state of the art. A surmise put forward after the data have been inspected does not have to meet any such demand and may be little more than a rationalization of them. Furthermore, such a surmise (which is, in fact, an interpretation of what has already happened) leads almost inevitably to conceptual gerrymandering. It cannot be falsified by the data from which it derives its structure.

Example 7.14. If I have a theory to account for the shape of the head of the human femur, then unless it is a hopelessly inept theory, it cannot be disproved by the facts on which it is based; and if it is not to be the subject of further enquiry, it cannot then be turned into a scientific theory.

This difficulty of surmisal after the data presents one of the major problems in trying to make a sound scientific theory out of Darwinian evolution. In principle, at least, all the "predictions" that any such theory could lead to are all matters of knowable fact; and whenever a scientist claims to "predict" what will be found when such-and-such data are collected, there is no way of being sure that he did not know what the empirical data showed before he made his prophesy and was gerrymandering conceptually. To be fair, one must recognize that much the same objection applies to astrophysics.

One way of looking at this line of reasoning is that surmise after the fact is not very sporting. It smacks of prophesy after the event. The surmise is not really advancing beyond the facts. And of course there is no corroboration except by the next experiment in which the same problem will again arise. On the other hand, if the present one were the last experiment possible (for instance, because a line of enquiry was made illegal, or a disease such as smallpox had become extinct), we might be forgiven for not wanting to take chances with it, even if we are left with uneasy doubts about how far we have discovered truth and how far we have merely done a rather complex Rorschach test or written a smooth epitaph to data.

The Nature of Pure Chance

Yet once again, we come to the question of questions. What do we make of the "pure chance" that is put up as an alternative to the notion of message? If this chance is what the probabilist seems to suppose and is of itself all the explanation that there is, then I see no problems of classical statistical interpretation. The proof is exactly what it purports to be, a probabilistic one. A causeless source of random variation, independent of any mechanism, may indeed produce a false pattern. If, on the other hand, this "pure chance" is merely a wasteland of ignorance and if we could account for all the data by specifying the causes if only we knew enough, then it is not at all clear what we mean by saying that this chance (which then means no more than we-know-not-what) could generate a *false* pattern. I suppose that we might mean that if ignorance may create the illusion of chance, it may also create false patterns; but what then allows us to decide that the pattern we read into unexplained data is false and not true? What is wrong with making a larger pattern out of smaller patterns? We do not say that the human body is an illusion because it is an assembly of parts with individual properties. The argument seems to say that our perception is the whole time assailed by false leads and only when the assault by one of these false leads is big enough to rise above the general clutter of false leads do we believe that what we perceive is truth. I am not at all sure whether that last statement makes any sense; but I find it difficult to imagine how it is to be cast in terms that we may manipulate formally. The reader will perceive that if I were deprived of the notion of pure chance, I would have no idea how we could make sense out of scientific data. I am not issuing an ultimatum; but I take no responsibility for resolving the difficulties of those who will insist right from the start that ultimately every component of what we observe can be accounted for in deterministic fashion.

Hypothesis and Design

Once we accept the idea that (rightly or wrongly) we are reading patterns into data, the question arises how far it is proper to do so. If one hypothesis made out of the facts gives a good fit, perhaps another, more elaborate hypothesis will fit even better. Indeed, in principle we can usually devise a model that will fit the data perfectly; but in general we will find that in doing so we have invoked as many structures (mainly parameters) in the model as we have data points. It is rather like converting more and more of the water in a swimming pool into ice cubes, until there is nothing left for them to float in. In the process, the model-fitting has succeeded brilliantly at a technical level but has failed totally in the scientific endeavor. For nothing has been simplified; nothing has been generalized; we have tested nothing and ventured nothing. We have replaced a set of twenty data by an equation containing twenty parameters. The obvious safeguard against this dismal outcome is to decide on the complexity of the problem in advance and to make sure that the number of data points far exceeds the number of parameters.

Nevertheless, in the last paragraph something very important has been left out of the whole discussion. As I have hinted, we have sacrificed our scientific goal to pure technique of proof. It illustrates what will be a recurrent theme in the last section of this book.

Neither proof nor certainty is enough.

The richness of science lies in the fact that *it is about something*. We shall see examples of statements that can be proved up to the hilt and mean virtually nothing ("All quadrupeds have four legs"); and statements very rich in meaning that are almost impossible to prove ("Love is the desire to enrich the being of another"). If I were forced to subsist on a diet of the one kind of statement or the other I would certainly pick those with meaning rather than those that were certain. Nevertheless, a scientist would hope for both proof (which is a *criterion* of understanding) and meaning (which is an *objective* of understanding). It is not easy to keep both goals in mind and in the right proportion during an era that has been cheapened by the idea that the main object of medical knowledge is a narrow definiteness. Only thus can one explain the supercilious attitude of so many physicians to fields such as human psychology, values, and esthetics, on the grounds that because they cannot furnish the excruciatingly exact measurements of physics, they are therefore intellectually beneath contempt.

PROBLEMS

7.1. If, in the nature of things, a proposition can be neither proved to be false, if false (i.e., it does not meet the assumption of falsifiability), nor to be true, if true (i.e., it does not meet the assumption of verifiability), then proof is an incompetent criterion of whether the proposition is sound. We must look elsewhere for our assurance. Where?

7.2. Suppose that blood pressure follows a Gaussian distribution. Then, as we know, it is exhaustively described by its mean and variance. A drug used to raise the blood pressure in the treatment of shock following car accidents gives the following results. The blood pressure before use has a mean of 75 mm Hg and a variance of 90 mm^2 Hg. The mortality rate is 25 percent. Among survivors, the mean blood pressure rises to 100. Thus, since the blood pressure in those that die is zero, the overall mean blood pressure after treatment is $(100)(3/4)$

+ (0)(1/4) = 75. Therefore, the treatment has had no effect on the mean of the blood pressure, and we conclude that it has no effect at all. Examine this argument carefully. Is it sound? Are you quite sure?

7.3. By an extension of the foregoing argument, suppose that only a small proportion of patients die and in the rest there is a considerable variation in responsiveness to a treatment, so that the overall mean and variance are unchanged. Would the interpretation put forward to explain the statistical findings in 7.2 still hold? If not, why not? If yes, are there any circumstances under which it would not apply?

7.4. How could we explore the question of whether women feel pain more or less than men do? Does this question have any meaning? Does the question have any ethical implications?

7.5. "Entropy (i.e., disorder) tends to a maximum." What would this statement mean if the universe were strictly deterministic, that is, that in principle every event could be exactly predicted if its antecedents were fully known?

7.6. If we accept that random components are causeless, what empirical (e.g., biological) meaning can we attach to correlation (that is, a presumably causal relationship) between the random components of two variables?

7.7. Which of the following processes do you perceive as deterministic, random, chaotic, autochthonous?
   a. The evasive action of a hare chased by a greyhound
   b. The song of the mockingbird
   c. Dreams
   d. The writing of poetry
   e. Sighing, hiccoughing, snoring

8 | The Structure of Medical Ideas

I shall start with two deeply rooted, and I believe sound, ideas of traditional medicine.

First, it is supposed that there exist disturbances of well-being that it is our responsibility as clinicians to understand, identify, prevent, anticipate, and treat. These disruptions we call anomalies, disorders, or diseases, loosely according to their gravity and prognosis. (This way of looking at an underlying disturbance asks us to accept some principle of unity, of individuation. There are a variety of such unities that one might appeal to, and a major task of this chapter is to say something about them.) It is argued that the clinician should not merely contend with these disturbances but should also aim to promote their opposites, by cultivating health and by encouraging the healthy and the well-endowed to reproduce rather than the unfit. These arguments are, on the whole, well received. However, one should realize the dangers and difficulties involved. Identifying what the optimal is that we are to encourage is often (and unwittingly) a matter of personal opinion.

Second, it is held that for the most part, clinicians, at least, do not come in direct contact with these disturbances but have to infer them indirectly from evidence, from what can be found by taking a history, by physical examination, from special tests (that are limited by current knowledge, by what is lawful, and other factors), and from noting the pattern and evolution of the disorder and its response to treatment. These limitations are only too familiar to the veterinarian, who is denied the patient's history.

While the foregoing is, in broad terms, sound, it is oversimplified. It glosses over difficulties at both stages. As we shall see, the first statement does not give due emphasis to the difficulty of defining where tolerable, even highly desirable, variation leaves off and anomaly begins. The second statement involves the hidden assumption that every problem the clinician encounters corresponds to something in the domain of disease. To sound out these difficulties, this chapter will be devoted to an illustrated enquiry. The problems will be approached in two ways. We shall begin with analysis: taking what it is that the clinician deals with and trying to reduce it to the underlying mechanisms. The second part, synthesis, starts with the basic causes and procedes, as if deductively, from them. We might use, as an image of the physician and the basic scientist, two teams of engineers making a tunnel through a mountain, starting from opposite sides and hoping to meet in the middle. There should be some sobering fear that they may not meet exactly, perhaps never meet at all; and there is something to be learnt on both sides from failures as well as successes.

On both sides.

We have suffered more than enough from the idea that the clinician is the student and somebody called the basic scientist is the teacher who is, sometimes patiently, sometimes scornfully, marking his homework exercises. Certainly, the basic scientist must police the clinician. But conversely, the clinician has at least two ways in which he can police the basic medical scientist. First he is in touch with not only a whole patient, but a living one; and one needs little biology to know that the whole is much more than the algebraic sum of the parts. Second, the clinician, if he is willing to listen and observe, can study what the patient's perspective is, which has as much right to be heard, and (from the humanist's viewpoint at least) has just as much meaning, as the physicist's or the mathematician's selective view of what the patient has. There is something to the idea that the problem is what the patient says it is, and not merely what may engage the interest of the purist. The clinician, without in any way being anti-intellectual, must guard against being overawed by the basic scientist to the point of riding roughshod over his patient.

ANALYSIS

It will be useful to work systematically through a series of clinical pronouncements, which start at the most superficial and end at the most penetrating that we have. I trust that the pattern we are following will rapidly become clear.

Let me suggest a simple mechanical model to be kept in mind throughout. Suppose that observers are standing outside a thick, more or less firm, hollow sphere (fig. 8.1). What they can see is the

A

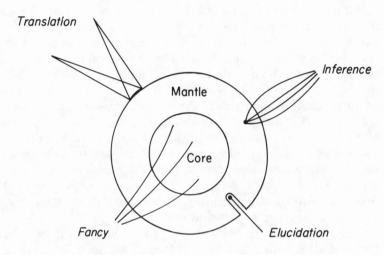

B

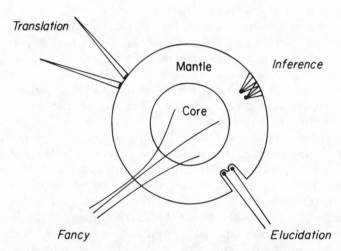

Figure 8.1. The terrestrial model of disease. *A:* One disease present. *B:* Two diseases present. Findings may be manifestly related to one event; there is no diagnostic problem to solve; and all that the clinician contributes is identification and translation (e.g., noting that there is simply a broken bone, or loss of body hair, or certain skin diseases, or scoliosis). Because of the immediateness, it is easy to tell one disease *A* from two *B*. If the findings are not obvious and diagnosis depends on indirect inference (e.g., the significance of breathlessness), it may not be so easy to say whether there is one disease or two. Elucidation may then require invasive procedures (represented in the analogy by mineshafts); even so, the mineshaft may not get close enough to the origin to say whether there is one disease or more. One must always bear in mind that a group of findings may be unrelated and all trivial. Any diagnosis is then pure fancy.

surface only, and they must make all their inferences from there. There are three essential parts: the *surface;* the solid part, or *mantle;* and the interior, or *core,* which is filled with gas or other fluid. It may strike the reader that this is like the geologist's model of the earth, and the analogy may prove such a useful one that I shall refer to it as the terrestrial model. The clinician may be seen as like the observer on the outside (or the geologist).

The symptoms and signs in the patient emanate from any or all of the three sites: the surface, the mantle, and the core. If we can see or infer that they arise from a single, compact cluster of points, all touching, we may regard this cluster as a disease entity. The physical aggregation is what gives it coherence; it is its own principle of unity. In the fluid central core the points freely and continually mix and do not form stable aggregates; thus, here this principle of unity is denied us, and there would be no purpose in looking for aggregates, which do not exist.

The clinician presented with symptoms and signs has to try to find out where they are coming from. They may be from one compact form in or on the mantle and may constitute what we call a disease; or from *several* foci in or on the mantle (several diseases); or they may be coming from random and unrelated particles (in the core) that furnish him with nothing that he can understand or deal coherently with, because they reflect no coherence.

We do not assume that all clusters in or on the mantle are diseases; but they may have manifestations that overlap with those of diseases, especially in the early stages. Thus, the clinician is caught up in two kinds of activities.

First, given a set of observations, he tries to see whether useful coherence may be read into them. This process, which we shall discuss in detail, is represented in the top half of figure 8.1.

Second, he has to distinguish two or more sources that may give rise to manifestations that, however, are not at once perfectly distinguishable. At times only one of the interpretations of the findings is coherent. It may be a matter of distinguishing, not between disease *A* and disease *B,* but between *A* and a chance mixture of findings, unrelated to each other, and each of them, taken separately, having an import. This process is shown in the bottom half of figure 8.1.

Now let us deal with a series of such patterns.

Surface Translation

Sometimes the clinical process may lie almost wholly on the surface and call for little or no analysis (fig. 8.1). Many terms in clinical use translate, without in any way changing, what the patient complains of. "Loss of appetite" or "being off one's food" is translated as *anorexia;* "itching" as *pruritus;* "ringing in the ears" as *tinnitus;* "sweating" as *diaphoresis;* and so on. It is hard to see what is gained by this, often pompous, kind of translation. Contrary to what many seem to suppose, a person is in no way a better clinician for knowing that *pernio* means chilblain (a disorder just as puzzling in Latin as in English) or that *microtia* means that the ear lobes are small. For my part, I use the so-called technical term if it is the shorter; otherwise, the English. Sometimes a crude term like "lump" (instead of *tumor*) or "heartburn" (instead of *pyrosis*) is the more useful. One of my orthopedic teachers used to say that if we talk about "breaking a thigh" rather than "fracturing a femur," we may perhaps remember that the damage includes tissues other than the bone, each calling for proper treatment in its own right.

In the terrestrial model, this pattern corresponds to finding some structure entirely on the surface and giving it a name; a dell, or a cliff, or a river. One can scarcely go wrong in saying that it is there, whatever language one puts it in. It does not usually help us much. On the other hand, it may prevent oversights.

Example 8.1. It does not call for much finesse to determine that a patient has six fingers (*hexadactyly*), and even the most obtuse patients are likely to notice it. Often it is one isolated finding and has no importance (except to those patients doing mental arithmetic in the decimal scale). But also it may be part of a more sinister disorder, such as the Ellis van Creveld syndrome (48) in which dwarfism and atrial septal defect—a form of congenital heart disease ("blue baby")—are common.

Example 8.2. Likewise, an iris may show patches of differing colors. This fact is well known to color photographers, who are none the worse for not knowing that it is called *anisochromia*. Again, it is commonly an isolated finding and harmless. But also it may be part of a more serious condition, such as the Waardenburg syndrome in which severe deafness is common (14).

Simple Esthetic Judgments

At times the clinician will add to the simple statement of the patient some features that involve judgments, either about what the patient thinks ("I am very ugly") or what the physician thinks (about, say, the patient's size or gracefulness). These additions may or may not help in diagnosis or management; but perhaps their main importance is that they may prove distractions from the matter in hand and may, consciously or unconsciously, modify the clinician's judgment. At any rate, they are no longer within the domain of simple, unmodified fact. Even if it may have no meaning to the geologist, to call one rock formation ugly and another a beauty spot has importance to the travel agent, and the tourists may influence how rapidly it changes.

Edited Translation

Sometimes the raw material needs to be cleaned up before it is translated.

Example 8.3. Even sophisticated people find it hard to describe a pain. They are apt to suppose that pain has location and quantity, even duration; but the quality of the pain often eludes them altogether.* Nevertheless, it may be of the utmost importance to the clinician whether the pain is steady, throbbing, momentary, smooth, stabbing, etc. But we all have at least a rough idea of what pain is.

Often, however, it is difficult to find out what the patient is complaining of.

Example 8.4. A patient will say "I have numbness in my back." *The back* includes any part of the patient that he cannot see without a mirror; and on questioning, most patients cannot say what part they are referring to without pointing to it; even then they may wave their hands vaguely. *Numbness* is used of an astonishing variety of states that are to be variously translated as loss, diminution, or perversion of feeling or loss of strength; sometimes it means stiffness, sometimes a vague discomfort or some other feature that defies analysis. There are many such symptoms that need to be carefully edited before being translated into dog Latin. Some patients float in fanciful similes ("It is like having a rat gnawing through your stomach") or hypothetical experiences which they fancy the doctor must have experienced ("You know what it's like when your heart turns to stone").

Interpretation into Symptom Complexes

This activity is more sophisticated and probably runs rather deeper. By a *symptom complex,* we mean a set of symptoms that are not merely haphazard but are found together disproportionately often and have a joint meaning that, taken separately, they do not have. I say that it probably runs deeper because a sophisticated

---

*Clinical students may gain insight from trying to describe to each other the characteristics of pains that they themselves have felt.

arrangement and interpretation of edited facts may be neither illuminating nor true. Nevertheless, nothing ventured, nothing gained. While recognizing some pattern is not enough to prove that we have a deeper understanding, it is certainly a necessary condition. We cannot understand something unless we have at some stage thought about it. But our evidence that the symptom complex exists is often subtle. Typically, there is no bedrock by which the truth is to be judged.

Example 8.5. Let us consider migraine.* In its most characteristic form, this condition is quite distinctive. I do not suppose that many neurologists doubt that it is a true entity. But in the present state of our knowledge at least, it is mainly a clinical definition and diagnosis. Blood chemistry will tell us nothing about it, nor will radiological examination. Necropsy (which in the terrestrial model is like sinking an exploratory mineshaft) provides no distinctive findings and is certainly a drastic turn in the diagnostic process. Should there be a dispute between two clinicians in an individual case, they may seek further opinions that may be more or less competent and experienced; but there is no gold standard to decide which is right. These difficulties are not to say that migraine is a fantasy, or that the diagnosis is worthless. We have a strong suspicion that the disturbance is coming from a focus in the mantle (so to speak) which we cannot reach directly as we could a skin lesion. But it is prudent to regard the diagnosis as provisional. When we understand better what is going on, we may conclude that what we call migraine may be, not one disorder, but several distinct conditions; and one of them may prove to be the same disorder as (say) bilious attacks or allergy or a form of epilepsy.

That this latter kind of regrouping is not merely a fantasy is readily illustrated from the past. What used to be called "dropsy" is now known to be a group of quite different disorders. What used to be thought of as separate diseases of the nervous system are now lumped together as "motor neurone disease."

Example 8.6. Consider the four conditions

1*a*. Lung cancer	1*b*. Pulmonary tuberculosis
2*a*. Metastasis* to the spine	2*b*. Pott's disease of the spine

---

*Migraine (hemicrania) is a type of headache, often severe, recurring on either side of the head but never both at once. It is often heralded by visual disturbances, accompanied by nausea, and aggravated by even moderately strong light. It is relieved or prevented by specific drugs. Newer means of diagnosis include studies on blood flow.

Metastasis means blood-borne spread of a cancer to a distant site.

In the early nineteenth century the two conditions 1*a* and 1*b* were probably not often distinguished, in unsophisticated clinical practice at least; likewise, 2*a* and 2*b* might have been regarded as more or less the same. On the other hand, the disorders of the lungs in the first line would be readily distinguished from the disorders of the back in the second. Today we see 1*a* and 2*a* as being closely related and also 1*b* and 2*b;* and we would regard those in the first column as quite different from those in the second. We are now thinking more in terms of pathology and less of anatomy. But I would not mortgage the future by saying that this perspective is the last word on the topic. It may be (for instance) that a genetic predisposition, or some peculiarity of the blood flow, determines whether the spine is susceptible to what in each case is secondary involvement in a blood-borne disease that may become generalized. The analogy here would be that what the geologist, on the surface, groups as part of the same process, depends on how he understands or believes the underlying rock to be orientated.

Canonization of an Arbitrary Criterion

Here, what the clinicians are doing is much more confidently identified as a diagnosis, but still with reservations. The clinician may be quite content from the standpoint of management to attach a label to a patient, but without requiring that the label means anything beyond the evidence on which it is given.

Example 8.7. If this sounds very complicated, let us start at once with a pointed question. Would the reader rather have an average blood pressure of 160/100 and be hypertensive, or one of 200/130 and be normotensive?*

Readers will fall into two groups. The first will answer yes or no. The second will say the question is absurd (fig. 8.2).

The first group believes there is a disorder, hypertension, of which high blood pressure is merely a manifestation—a useful, but fallible, sign, as cough is in bronchitis. To say it is fallible means that diagnosis from the blood pressure alone will from time to time lead to misclassification. Thus the figure 200/130 mm Hg may be really from the normotensive population, but an unusually high reading for it, and conversely for the figure of 160/100. Those who have answered *no* think that it is the hypertension that matters to prognosis, not the blood pressure itself; and those who answer *yes* believe the opposite. And we could make a case for either viewpoint.

*The reader should try to answer this question before reading on.

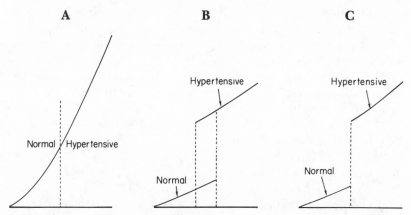

Figure 8.2. Three possible interpretations of the notion of hypertension. On the vertical axis is represented the damage done as a function of the level of the blood pressure, which is shown on the horizontal axis. *A:* The cost may increase smoothly with the blood pressure: there is no natural breakpoint and the definition is purely arbitrary. *B:* There may be two underlying states with some overlap in the blood pressure levels they produce, and which is therefore a fallible sign of the underlying state. *C:* There may be a critical breakpoint at which the prognosis suddenly deteriorates to a degree that dwarfs the ordinary systematic impact of level of blood pressure.

Readers who say that the question is absurd (not trivial, but absurd) clearly believe that there is nothing behind the blood pressure that merits being called hypertension: that *hypertension* is merely a word that we use to mean high blood pressure. The two terms bear exactly the same relationship to each other that *itching* and *pruritus* do. It is a surface translation of the findings. Such people might say that Jones is very hypertensive but Brown is even more hypertensive. The first group, however, would have to decide whether a person is hypertensive or not.

Example 8.8. Women are heterozygous for hemophilia or not. No physician would ever say that Mary is very heterozygous but Peggy is even more heterozygous. The most that they would say is that Mary is very likely to be heterozygous and Peggy even more likely to be. Any degrees are attached, not to the underlying state, but to the strength of the evidence on which we infer it.

In our terrestrial analogy we have a corresponding rivalry. The reply of readers in the first group is like arguing that it is wiser to build a house in one state than in another, in view of the housing laws. The boundaries of the states (even if they are arbitrary) are perfectly definite and represent surface markings, and the jurisdiction of laws corresponds exactly to them. The reply of those in the second group is like arguing about building a house in a site free of earthquakes. Earthquakes are commoner and more severe in California than in Oregon. So the state is still something of a guide; but it is not really the issue. The earthquakes originate below the surface, and neither their origins nor their effects stop abruptly at the state boundaries. It is arguably better to live in California than to die in an earthquake in Oregon.

If this distinction is now clear, we may address quickly a number of classes of these ambiguous ideas.

Metricated (Measured) Traits. Together with hypertension, we might put under this grouping obesity, tallness, glaucoma, dwarfism, hyper . . . emia (many kinds). In many cases, there are undoubtedly some underlying diseases that produce abnormalities of these measurements. The unifying principle here is quantity.

Example 8.9. Obesity may be caused by hypothalamic disease and by trisomy 21. However, the key diagnosis in such cases is not obesity but what this underlying disorder is. Obesity is thought of as a feature or even a well-known complication of a disease. The absence of obesity is not to be taken as proof positive that the patient does not have trisomy 21, for instance.

Artificially Metricated Traits. The argument here is much the same as in the foregoing, but the scale is not altogether objective or universally accepted (as measurements in the physical system of centimeter-gram-seconds or their equivalents are); instead it is put together by giving arbitrary scores to arbitrarily chosen data. Measurements of intelligence, mood, fantasy life, etc., are made by constructing and trying out a series of tests and then finding a system of scoring the answers that in some sense has meaning.

Genetic Diseases. At least some genetic diseases have little unifying warrant except that, however ill-defined, they are inherited generation after generation without losing any of their force. Von Willebrand's disease is of this type (49); so perhaps are dyslexia (50) and familial polyposis of the colon (14, 18). The fact of an inheritance that is conserved argues some underlying factor that is behaving like a causal unity. This argument is not necessarily the same as saying that there is a specific gene involved. That claim for the diseases mentioned is at least in formal doubt; and in a balanced translocation, it is certainly not true that a single gene only is at fault. It is the two facts of nonindependence in the features *and* the pattern of transmission that makes the claim so convincing. Repeated earthquakes detected in various locales and always, or nearly always, with the same findings, suggest to us that there are multiple foci that may be related to each other (by the San Andreas fault for example).

Syndromes. As a generalization of the foregoing, if there is a set of findings that occur together more often than could be explained by chance, and if there is good reason for believing that they are not all the same finding in various disguises or that the one leads causally to the other, then we have evidence that there is an underlying disease entity at work. This idea is somewhat elusive and needs to be looked at a little more carefully. First, the evidence of (nonrandom) association calls for serious attention to the reference population.

Example 8.10. Sickle-cell disease and favism both occur frequently in West Africans. If the reference population is *all human beings,* the joint occurrences of these two diseases will be a true association resulting from a high concentration of both in one group; if the reference population is *West Africans,* there may very well not be any association. There is, to our knowledge, no causal connection between them pathogenetically, since sickle-cell disease and favism are controlled at different and unlinked genetic loci. The causal connection where the reference set is *all human beings* is an evolutionary one: the fact is that both disorders affect red blood cells and are thus believed to give some protection against malaria; hence both are selected for in malarious environments.

• *The notion of a syndrome requires that the features occur nonindependently (more commonly than we would expect by chance) in any and every nontrivially defined population.**

Note, however, that if the traits are never separable at all, we may be led to suspect a tautology. ("The right leg is shorter than the left" and "the left leg is longer than the right" are not mutually corroborative statements.)

The second issue to which we must pay attention is that the *less* likely the features are to occur together by chance if unrelated, the more evidence they furnish of a significant relationship if they occur together; and conversely, the commoner they are, the more significant it is that they should not occur together.

Example 8.11. Imagine a prospector looking for radium with a Geiger counter. There will be some scattered random noise under any casual circumstance. If a high counting rate is found in one period of counting and in one place, it may be explained in three broad ways. First, it may be due to chance. (The longer it persists,

---

*By a nontrivially defined population, I mean one that would make such an association possible. *A* and *B* cannot possibly be associated in a population *defined* by the fact that it does not have any variation in trait *B*, for instance. We cannot look for evidence of an association between age and blood pressure in a group of men who are all celebrating their twenty-fifth birthdays.

the less plausible this explanation is.) Second, it may mean that there is a concentrated deposit of radium that will be worth mining. Third, it may mean that there is radium, but it is so scattered as not to be worth special effort on the part of the prospector. Nevertheless, the sanitary officer may consider diffusely scattered radium just as dangerous to life as if there were a single concentrated deposit.

In the analogy, the clinician may perceive a symptom, sign, or other finding as a random aberration of no importance. It may come from a sharply defined source that should be remedied. It may be so inextricably interwoven in the whole personality as to be beyond cure.

Example 8.12. Everybody is tired at one time or another, perhaps following hard work, perhaps for no clear reason. A patient who is persistently tired may have a particular disorder that can, and should, be remedied, such as Addison's disease, myxedema, or anemia. However, some are "born tired"—they may have personalities in which enthusiasm of any kind has no part. To alter the latter may call for action so radical that it might amount to a new formation of the personality, which in its extreme form would involve the deepest moral, legal, and political issues.

Example 8.13. Suppose that a child's performance in school falters. Perhaps the cause is a brief lapse of attention. Perhaps it is due to an early brain tumor. It may be that the child is less intelligent than average. The first should be ignored; the second, treated; the third, accepted with compassionate understanding and hope.

However, what of the diagnostic problem of deciding among these three explanations for a set of symptoms or signs?

There are hundreds of minor disorders (wax in the ears, sweaty palms, a few pimples, some gray hairs, etc.) likely to occur among the otherwise healthy. They will tend to assemble randomly, and in any patient we might expect four or five of them together. That fact is of no significance. On the other hand, several of them may occur as a manifestation of serious disease. How is one to distinguish probabilistically? It depends on the circumstances. The findings might come to light:

1. In a symptomless patient examined for some totally other reason (say, a routine annual examination), our tendency will be to think that with respect to these traits he is a random sample from his class.
2. Three of the abnormal findings may be discovered in a di-

rected search prompted by the fourth. The association is then likely to mean business precisely because the search is directed.

3. If the examination is due to the symptoms (that is, the enquiry is started by the patient), we can no longer treat him as random with respect to them. The conjunction is even less likely to be significant than in 1, above.* Any anxious patient can always assemble a group of such commonplace, and often trivial, findings. The fact that the patient has consulted the doctor may tell much more about the patient than about any disease. The actual symptoms may be no more (but also no less) important than those words the patient uses to describe them.

Example 8.14. Consider the following findings. *A.* The patient's feet are cold in damp weather. *B.* He does not have athlete's foot. *C.* He has no hair on the back of his toes. They are all common states, and each in itself is quite harmless. But let us now look at them in three kinds of circumstances.

1. The physician discovers them in a patient who has come complaining that every time he walks a hundred yards or more he has a severe pain in his calves that makes him stop. They are all confirmatory signs of a diagnosis that has been suggested by the pain: intermittent claudication (i.e., arterial narrowing), a condition related to angina pectoris (q.v.).
2. They are found in a female patient on routine examination for a job. They should be ignored.
3. A 35-year-old marathon runner who comes to the physician worried because of them is probably looking for something to attach his anxiety to and is in need of psychotherapy.

If the clinician finds a number of rare features in a patient, he may feel that their concurrence by chance is an implausible explanation. Then he may be able to trace them to a single clear focus—say, a pneumonia or a brain tumor or perhaps a disturbance of some bodily system as in the Marfan syndrome. There may or may not be a specific treatment.

Depending on the features, the disease may be far from the

---

*More generally, wherever features are the reason for any encounter, it may be impossible to explore associations with them. The clinician is often concerned about patients that die unexpectedly, because he expects most of his patients to live. He may have fears that some major disorder was overlooked clinically. But the morbid anatomist may be curious, but hardly concerned that his subjects have died: he expects those coming to necropsy to be dead.

surface, so that the process of diagnosis is remote and heavily inferential. Such is the case in most neurological problems.

Example 8.15. If the patient says he has right-sided blindness, for instance, the neurologist will test to see whether one *eye* is blind or one *visual field* is blind (a distinction that few patients make unless prompted). If the latter, the lesion lies behind the optic chiasma. If the pupillary reflexes are intact, the lesion must lie beyond the brain stem. And so on.

Example 8.16. At the other extreme in acute physical trauma there may be almost no inference involved. There is nothing to puzzle out about the cause of death in a man who has been instantaneously killed in a bomb explosion. It is purely academic which particular bones were broken. In the same way, the problems with a child who has been scalded by a kettle of boiling water lie in assessment and treatment; but it takes little finesse to know what has happened or to decide from the history whether it is a single incident of scalding. But the fact that the diagnosis of scalding is transparent does not make it in any sense a more shallow or a less satisfactory diagnosis. To the contrary, in clarity it is vastly superior to a diagnosis like peptic ulcer or rheumatoid arthritis, where both the diagnostic process is more difficult and the diagnosis that is made is hazier—with arbitrary limits and at best an uncertain cause.

SYNTHESIS

Hitherto, we have been concerned with what are, or appear to be, significant problems in medicine and have attempted to break them down into their component parts; hence, we try to decide which of them are real problems and which figmented, and how they might be cast into a more useful form. One can quote famous examples (from infectious disease or vitamin deficiencies) in which this analytical method has worked admirably. There is no better example than retrolental fibroplasia (51) at a purely clinical level, or pernicious anemia (52) at a biochemical one.

There is another approach that can be viewed as the very opposite of analysis (or dissecting into components), where the stimulus to enquiry is not a problem to be resolved into parts but a set of facts to be built up. The distinction may be nicely illustrated from modern microbiology.

Example 8.17. When Legionnaires' disease came to medical attention, in time it became clear that it was infectious; and the great *analytical* achievement was to convert the rather nebulous clinical picture into a precise form as the manifestation of a specific organism, *Legionella pneumophila* (53).

Example 8.18. The *synthetic* counterpart is the orphan virus, a type of organism that, it is felt, must have clinical significance but with which no defined disease has been associated so far.

Again, nucleic acids and their metabolites were soon enough incriminated by analysis as at least an underlying cause of gout; but it was only much more slowly that it was perceived (by conceptual synthesis) that this pervasive group of compounds, the nucleic acids, function as the embodiments of genetic data.

Now it is a mistake, and a very common one, to suppose that all the problems of medical science can be solved by the analytical or the synthetic approach alone, to the exclusion of the other. It would be false to imagine that the clinician has no need of the biochemist; but on the other hand, one merely has to think of the management of fractures to see that the biochemist alone could not meet anything like all the needs of medicine. There is nothing whatsoever to be gained by foolish rivalries between these two complementary approaches. The complementarity may be conveniently discussed by addressing the relationship between two perspectives of the pathologist.

ETIOLOGY AND PATHOGENESIS

The issues are clarified by comparing the meaning and scope of two terms.

Etiology

Etiology (literally, "the science of causes") is concerned with discovering the characteristics and circumstances of those people who are apt to suffer from particular diseases. Common nonspecific etiological features that are traditionally looked at are age, sex, race, occupation, diet, organisms, genes, toxins, and so forth. When one of them becomes incriminated, the nature of the relationship may be successively refined until perhaps it is precisely pinpointed.

Example 8.19. In sickle-cell anemia, for instance, the successive steps included

1. Recognition of a particular form of anemia, common among Negroes.
2. Discovery that, when deprived of oxygen, their red cells assume an odd shape.

3. Demonstration that their hemoglobin is distinguishable by electrophoresis from the normal type, and
4. Isolation of an abnormal peptide fragment on fingerprint analysis
5. That proved to be due to an explicit amino acid substitution
6. Traceable to an anomalous nucleotide.

Step 5, completed in 1959, was the supreme analytic triumph, the model goal of etiology (54). One could make much the same kind of claim for aneurin deficiency in beriberi (55), Koch's bacillus in tuberculosis (56), and HMG coenzyme A reductase deficiency in familial hypercholesterolemia (57).

However, we may wonder what the clinician is to do with the foregoing reduction. He will find that somewhat complex changes in his focus have gone on as the analysis has proceeded. For one thing, each step in the investigation has more or less subtly distorted the questions with which he started.

The nineteenth century physician's concern with "consumption" has shifted to the study of tuberculosis, which will now exclude as irrelevant much of what he started with (e.g., other causes of cavitation of the lungs) yet will include much that he did not think of at all in this connection (e.g., lupus vulgaris or a certain type of meningitis). The systematic enquiry has profoundly changed both the diagnostic criteria and the definitions. The interrelations between these two features give rise to very slippery problems (see chapter 12). Obviously, the analytical identification of the fundamentals of tuberculosis paves the way for rational treatment.

Nevertheless, the analytical approach also has perils and disadvantages that in the flush of success have been overlooked, and at times with heavy penalties.

Example 8.20. Doubtless one can exclude the diagnosis of typhoid fever if the specific organism *S. typhi* is persistently absent. Indeed, this is trivially true if the presence of this organism is to be a *necessary criterion* of typhoid fever. However, that does not tell us how to interpret the fact that the organism may be found to be present in a symptomless patient. In order to sustain his etiological theory, the microbiologist has had to devise what are in truth face-saving terms like "chronic carriers." When I call them face-saving, I do not mean that the term *carrier* is not a useful one, or even a rather bold and illuminating new idea. All the same, it is a crack in any kind of etiological absolutism. Typhoid is not merely a matter of the organism; the host is also important. For one thing, insofar as science is concerned with replacing a large number of particular

instances with a small number of generalizations, the need to introduce such a term in order to preserve the splendid unifying idea of
S. *typhi* is a setback. The more qualifications that have to be added
to the original idea in order to keep it afloat, the more its claims on
our belief are weakened. There is clearly more to an infection than
the presence of the organism. If you please, S. *typhi* is a *necessary* but
not a *sufficient* cause for the disease. And the problem of how and
why a disease may sometimes, but not always, result from the operation of etiological factors is the study of pathogenesis.

The distinction is admirably illustrated in my own field of
genetics.

Example 8.21. Many talented scientists have shown the etiological
significance of specific factors in genetic disease, and the majority
of them have been basic scientists, many with a broad interest, but
no formal training, in clinical medicine. Many of them perhaps
suppose, because the precise etiology of sickle-cell disease is known,
that therefore the problem of sickle-cell disease is solved. This
supposition would be coldly received by the pathologist on whom
devolves the task of building the bridge between etiology and
clinical medicine. Meanwhile, the internist is as much in the dark as
ever as to why the concomitant clinical disorder takes the form it
does (sickle-cell crises, small-artery thrombosis, susceptibility to sal-
monella and pneumococcal infections, resistance to malarial infections, stunted growth, etc.).

With comparatively few exceptions, there has been virtually no
dialogue between the geneticist and the pathologist. I suspect that
the formidable problems of studying the genetics of systems may
explain why the geneticist has fought shy of the pathologist, the
anatomist, the physiologist, and the psychologist, all of whose interests are centered, not on basic traits, but on *systems*. But, as if
arguing that one might as well be hanged for a sheep as for a lamb,
some geneticists have attempted to grapple with entire and complex diseases: atherosclerosis, schizophrenia, and cancer; and they
have done so in two ways. Either they have refused all responsibility for anything but the genetics (as if the clinician's infallible and
unambiguous perception of disease did not need to be edited in the
light of genetics and genetical analysis at all) or they have regarded
atherosclerosis as if it is quite simply an inborn error of cholesterol
metabolism, and cancer nothing more than a somatic mutation.

Etiological Factors. In practice, the degree to which an etiological factor is resolved varies. Thus, a listing of such factors does
not necessarily consist of mutually exclusive items.

Example 8.22. It would be appropriate to list genes and chromosomes as separate etiological items, although chromosomes are groupings of genes. This duplication and overlap makes for rather untidy classifications. We may hope that when medical knowledge is good enough, we will fare much better. However, trends at the present time are doing little to foster this kind of coherence, as I shall try to illustrate.

The nearest scheme I can propose at the present time is that man exists as a genotype with a particular immune system, metabolism, and personality, in contact with, and largely expressing himself through, an environment. It is false to make a *division* of these etiological factors into "nature" and "nurture" or "genes" and "environment." That tack has been pursued extensively; and while it has not led to any crass absurdity, it has not led to any useful discoveries either. A little reflection will suggest why. For on the one hand, it involves the belief that this partition is exhaustive; and on the other hand, it has led to artificial and obscure ways of fitting certain factors into the scheme. Let us take the argument a little more slowly.

There are all manner of theoretical problems about the inner nature of causality. But here I shall leave them severely alone. At a robust, practical level, it is established that A causes B if, whenever by a *manipulation* independent of B (i.e., by intervening artificially), we cause A to happen or to change, then B happens or changes also. Whenever, for legal or other reasons, we are not in a position to produce or change A, then the evidence (noting how again B varies as A varies spontaneously) leads to conclusions that are rather weaker and need to be tempered with common sense and background knowledge. That statement, though naive, will do for the present.

Example 8.23. Two major factors put forward to account for what people are like (their *phenotypes*) are genetics and environment. If I should claim that genetic factors are related to height, I imply that by one method or another I have established that an *observed* variation in genes (G) produces a corresponding variation in height. The corresponding *observation* may be put forward that environmental factors (E) influence height. Without introducing either further assumptions or empirical data, I cannot argue that G and E between them determine the height in every particular. Nor do I personally believe that such is the case. However, a claim that genetic and environmental factors explain the height entirely has been kept alive by the rather contrived device of defining *environmental effects* to comprise everything that is not genetic; or by the less naive, but just as empty, ruse of introducing a third component, "interaction." We shall have more to say about this term later. Meanwhile, I would point to two further different kinds of factors that do not really fit into either *G* or *E*.

The third factor, involving the notion of randomness, is utterly incompatible with the notion of cause. As we have noted several times, to say that something is "random" may be to use a false term meaning that it is indeed caused, but the cause has not yet been identified. Some would say (on evidence that escapes me) that variation always has a cause. One instance that belies this claim in the genetic field is the current belief that the process of Lyonization (24), whereby one X chromosome in each cell is rendered inactive, is a purely random process. If this is so, it does not mean anything to say that the outcome is produced by genetic mechanisms, although its impact operates through them. In the same way, particle physics argues that disintegration of a radionuclide is causeless and what impact that may have on health is causeless, even if the channel through which it operates is environmental. But so far as we know, there is no prospect of manipulating either Lyonization or radioactive decay, and hence (by the stricter criteria) no prospect of establishing causation.

The fourth factor, which is much more difficult to grapple with and more controversial, is free will, an example of the autochthonous variation we discussed in chapter 7. It would be absurd for me to address in one paragraph the topic of whether or not there is such a thing as free will. The main support for the idea comes from introspection (which much Freudian psychology would dismiss as rationalization) and from the pragmatic yardstick of common sense. The whole conduct of clinical medicine is based on the assumption that it is at least sometimes within the power of at least some patients to cooperate or not with their treatment at least some of the time. Particle physics suggests the ultimate reduction of all action to definable cause is false; mathematics, that it may not be provable; probability theory, that it is unnecessary. Determinists would counter by saying that indeterminism is inelegant, scientifically pusillanimous, nonheuristic, and a betrayal of four hundred years of rigorous science. The question is not to be resolved by assertions alone, however fervent or vigorous. From a practical viewpoint, it would be mere obscurantism to treat the problem as if, from a scientific viewpoint, it were settled. My own (still tentative) opinion at the present time is that while most of what we observe from a physical standpoint can be described and at least tentatively explained by causes, there is an irreducible minimum of uncertainty.

The Notion of Interaction. Two lines of thought suggest that even if randomness and free will are illusory, in no kind of biological theory could one account altogether for all factors through either genetics or environment, acting in isolation from each other. There must be a further component, which has been given the title (unfortunately a confusing and ambiguous one) of *interaction*.

The first line of thought about interaction is biological: that certain events occur only when two causes come together.

Example 8.24. A certain kind of anemia (favism) occurs only when a patient with deficiency of the enzyme glucose-6-phosphate dehydrogenase takes certain drugs or eats certain foods. Either factor alone has no such effect. The genetic cause can express itself only in particular environments.

The second, formalistic, line of thought is that when one measures the amount of variation in the phenotype produced by genetic factors in a fixed environment and the amount produced by environmental factors in animals all with the same genotype, the sum of these two observed amounts proves not to be equal to the total observed variation of the phenotype. If there is a deficit, the statistician says there is a *positive interaction* (to make up the deficit), and conversely. If their sum is greater than the total variation, he calls it *negative interaction*. In neither case is the interaction observed: it is merely inferred by the hole in the equation.

I have said the term *interaction* is an unfortunate one, a view that becomes evident when we look at it more closely. A major problem arises because the two formulations, the biological and the formalistic, which are given the same name and seem to be saying the same thing, are not at all equivalent. Rather obviously, the notion of negative interaction has no biological meaning. Either two factors have some impact on each other or they do not. They cannot have less than no impact; so it is hard to see what we would mean by saying biological interaction is negative. If they are mutually antagonistic (as starvation and exercise are in the development of muscle), the biologist may restate the interaction in terms of a contrary to make the outcome mutually supportive. ("Appropriate food intake and exercise promote the development of muscle.") Moreover, if the dietary cholesterol and certain genes interact to influence the blood cholesterol level, we would also expect that they will continue to interact if we are thinking about them in some formalistically disguised terms (e.g., the logarithm of the blood level). In just the same way, the effect of a particular person being hit by a particular moving car on a particular occasion does not seem to depend on whether the physicist *measures* the kinetic energy or the momentum of the car—which are both germane, but not proportional quantities; neither does the meaning of a physical experiment depend on the native language of the investigator. On the other hand, what a statistician calls an interaction depends exquisitely on how the measurements are expressed. There is even a branch of statistics concerned with reformulating the data so as to get rid of an inconvenient interaction in the formalistic sense.

Example 8.25. In the laying down of bone, there is both a statistical and a chemical interaction between the concentrations of calcium ion and phosphate ion; there is still a chemical interaction between the *logarithms* of their concentrations; but it turns out that changing the measurements to their logarithms abolishes the statistical interaction. It is obvious that, seen from a statistical standpoint, what is called interaction may be purely a property of the terms of measurement. But this statement would have no biological or chemical meaning whatsoever. Readers who feel confused by these ideas are to be congratulated. It shows that they have some perception that there is confusion here. I hope that it will alert them to the ambiguous way words are used by those who make no real attempt to disentangle the issues.

Other Etiological Factors. As well as the major factors we have already mentioned (genome, environment, randomness, free will, interaction), we may mention two other groups of factors.

The first is *ecology,* or the relationship among species. The fact that the other species also have mechanisms inside them and each has its own urge to survive leads to peculiar dynamics that are quite different from those of a simple environment, and that have complicated and often paradoxical results.

Example 8.26. Sunlight is an environmental factor. It may harm the skin, which will respond in various ways. But our skin does not change the sunlight.

Example 8.27. However, man chasing game may make two discoveries. First, the game may fight back. Second, if he overhunts, he may eventually starve because of the scarcity of game. Man may die because he is too skilled a hunter. He may also die if he is an utterly inept hunter. The reward for skill is not monotonic.

The other factor is *society,* or man's relationship to his own kind. Again, the complexity of the dynamics (which in this case operates symmetrically among the components) means that society cannot be treated as an inert lump of environment. Even a little exploration will tell us that a society has very complicated properties that are not easily traceable to those of the individuals in it, and perhaps not to be explained in that way at all. In part, these properties arise because society is corporate. (Personal equality or inequality, for instance, is a property of a group and has no meaning in the isolated individual.) In part, they arise because a society has structures (e.g., the phenomena of leadership, specialization, politics). Anybody who has ever lived in a village where everybody knows everybody else and a stranger cannot pass unnoticed is aware of why the character of crime there is different from that in the anonymity of New York or London. One's ranges of acquaintance in the two societies are quite different. Society makes specialization possible; and the medicine, engineering, education, law, and religions to which they give rise have a profound impact on the pattern of disease.

Pathogenesis

I have not despaired that with sufficient knowledge and ingenuity we will be able to trace the relationship between the etiology and the disease itself; but this is no trivial undertaking. The details of what we know are within the purview of the pathologists, and I have no ambitions to usurp their function. Nevertheless, it does fall within my province to sketch the purely logical aspects of what the pathologist is about. A great deal of pathology has always been analytical rather than synthetic, and for two obvious reasons. The first reason comprises the constraints imposed by conscience. The experimental pathologist is always more or less reluctant to induce even a trivial disease in a human being; and the mere fact that a person is apparently rational and volunteers to be a subject in a study of artificially produced disease does not by any means dispose of all the moral problems. In particular, there is a special reluctance to accept as volunteers the young, the retarded, or the convicted criminal. Second, the other course—to use animals as subjects for experimentation—always raises doubts as to the relevance of such experiments to human beings. Certainly there are plenty of disruptions (such as infections, dietary manipulations, coagulation, brain injuries) that produce very different responses among species. The synthetic approach to the study of disease by experimental means must therefore be used with some caution.

It is not easy to communicate to those who have no grasp of pathology as a dynamic system how the complexities arise. But there are a number of factors that must be included in any equation of disease. First, the etiological factors will pass unnoticed if they are not in some measure disruptive; and, broadly, disruption tends to call forth compensating and corrective processes, collectively called homeostasis.* Where these countermeasures can do their work unobtrusively, we do not often use the term *disease*. But the patient may feel ill either because of the primary cause (to be stabbed in the chest is painful) or the body's reaction to it (as vomiting when poisoned or shivering when cold). The threshold at which malaise is felt may vary among subjects.

Example 8.28. Human beings sweat as a means of getting rid of heat. But some patients, for genetic (14) or other reasons, cannot sweat, and overheating is then a more serious problem.

Example 8.29. When one stands, the blood pressure tends to fall, and the blood vessels constrict in compensation. Sometimes this produces a momentary dizziness. In some patients, slowness in compensating may be severely incapacitating. In some, the response is inadequate, and fainting may occur.

Thus, it is not altogether clear where homeostasis leaves off and disease begins; and this indefiniteness will be something of a problem even in an acute disturbance. When the disruption continues and extends, the real business of pathology begins, and the destructive effect of the disease becomes mixed up with the combative and reconstructive forces of the body: inflammation, antibody formation, repair, regrowth, scarring, and the like. These combative forces, while overcoming the original sources of injury, may prove a mixed blessing. In doing its job in quinsy or diphtheria, inflammation may produce swelling and thus lead to obstruction of breathing; exuberant repair of destroyed tissues may be unsightly; scarring of the cornea may blind; and so forth. The arterial disease of middle life, atherosclerosis, may be due to the scarring that results in the repair of thrombosis; it may lead to further thrombosis; and so on in alternating episodes. Antibodies may become excessive and lead to allergies and so-called autoimmune disease. Scarring from the healing of a gastric ulcer may lead to death from starvation.

It is small wonder that analytical pathology is taxed when such diseases are studied late in their course. A necropsy may be more like archeology than the study of a dynamic process. Pathologists have devised all manner of ingenious methods of grappling with such puzzles. Yet they run into a problem of identifying the true

---

*This term was originally introduced by Cannon (58) to describe the restorative process identified by Claude Bernard (59). It has been metaphorically used in population genetics by Lerner (60) and in an ontogenic sense by Waddington (61). I use it here in Cannon's original sense.

nature of disease, for which there is no ready solution. I can perhaps illustrate the point with an example that has been of some
interest to me.

Example 8.30. For a century or more there has been much debate
as to the significance of certain collections of lipid that commonly,
perhaps usually, appear in the lining of the larger blood vessels,
even in childhood. Some see them as the earliest lesion of atherosclerosis and some as a finding of no importance at all. The dispute
is not as yet resolved (62), and it is not easy to see how it can be so
long as the data are to come from necropsies; for then there is
information available at one age only. One does not see the same
patient necropsied at various ages; and we have seen earlier the
perils of trying to make diachronic (serial) inferences from syn-
chronic (instantaneous or cross-sectional) data. Until such time as
repeated observations on the same person can be made by some
noninvasive technique *that we are quite sure causes no local damage to
the blood vessel,* our evidence must consist of statistical inferences
from populations rather than from studies on the dynamics of
individuals. There is, besides, an elusive dilemma for the pathologist. The earlier the lesions that he studies, the more uncomplicated they are and the easier to disentangle and interpret; but also
the less sure he is that they are truly part of the disease of interest.
The later the lesions, the more assured he is that what he is looking
at is authentic atherosclerosis, but the more confused the various
components of evidence. I suppose that the best course is some
kind of compromise between the two demands.

Example 8.31. Again, let us look at cancer of the bowel. It is
widely believed that cancers develop only in antecedent intestinal
polyps, that is, in plain Anglo-Saxon, warts in the gut. I have several times referred to genetic diseases in which such polyps are common (18, 27), and we have safe techniques (mainly colonoscopy) of
observing them repeatedly. Hence, in principle at least, we have
the means to do diachronic studies. The main obstacle is the lack of
precise landmarks in the gut and the difficulty of deciding whether
a polyp seen now is indeed the same polyp seen a year ago.

It is easy to see why in the face of such analytical problems there
has emerged a synthetic approach, experimental pathology, with
heavy reliance on experiments in animals. However, one should
not overlook the theoretical arm of synthetic pathology. This approach puts forward a model of the development of a disease.
Sometimes it is heavily mathematical, as in the models proposed by
Armitage and Doll (63), Moolgavkar et al. (64), and others, of the
process by which cancer develops; sometimes it is mainly genetic, as

in Knudson's model of retinoblastoma (65); sometimes it is mainly immunological, like many of the models of nephritis; and so forth. But in all such cases it is a matter of surmise based on reasonable evidence, which leads to predictions that can be tested. I must leave the details to the pathologist.

SYNTHETIC SEMIOLOGY

In discussing analysis, we saw in the geological model that the starting point of enquiry might be the signs and symptoms from which the clinician tries to delimit diseases, which are then scrutinized. In synthesis we may see the reverse process at work. Study of basic mechanisms may lead to tentative predictions that prompt the clinician to look for signs, even diseases, that have been hitherto overlooked.

Example 8.32. It was the study of bacteria that led Lister to realize that suppuration is a disease, and not an integral part of normal healing, as orthodox surgeons had taught up to that point.

Example 8.33. E. B. Wilson (66), actively searching for medical applications of Mendelian genetics, was able in 1911 to predict what patterns of inheritance might be expected, and hence imposed order on human color blindness.

Example 8.34. No doubt but that clinical cardiology (especially skill in auscultation and the interpretation of the venous pulse in the neck) has gained greatly from phonocardiography, echocardiography, and the polygraph.

Example 8.35. Finesse in the examination of the patient with hepatic failure has been spurred by an understanding of basic metabolism; and the same is true of endocrinology.

It is not difficult to imagine other instances of the same pattern; but in fact this activity has been not nearly popular enough in recent years, and perhaps there is still much to be discovered about what theoretical studies may do to the bedside acumen of the clinician.

PROBLEMS

8.1. Analyze what the meaning of the following common symptoms may be: (*a*) weakness, (*b*) indigestion, (*c*) dizziness, (*d*) lethargy.

8.2. Consider the problems in establishing the benefits of early preventive intervention in a chronic disease with a slow onset and development.

8.3. The only two inhabitants of an island were given the choice by the Boundary Commission of having their island become part of Vermont or of New Hampshire. One picked Vermont because the taxes are lower. The other picked New Hampshire because the climate there is milder. Consider the merits of these two approaches, and find analogous issues in medicine.

8.4. In identifying to which side a femur belongs, students may put together three pieces of information: the linear aspera is posterior; the greater trochanter is lateral; and the adductor tubercle is distal.

    a. Under what circumstances will (fallible) students assign the femur to the correct side? (Careful!)

    b. Let the proportions that get the three facts correct be A, B, and C, respectively. Assume all three guesses are independent. What average proportion of students will make the right assignment?

    c. What sound generalization might this argument lead to?

8.5. In Down's syndrome (trisomy 21, or mongolism) a regular feature is that the tongue is partly outside the mouth. Some hold that the tongue is too large, and others that the mouth is too small. Consider how one might decide between them, and suggest other profitable approaches.

8.6. Consider two variable human attributes, X and Y, each of which is just as likely be positive as negative. If both are positive or both negative, the results are concordant; otherwise, they are discordant. How would you biologically interpret concordance rates of 0 percent, 5 percent, 50 percent, 80 percent, and 100 percent?

9 | The Development of Medical Ideas

In this chapter, I am not attempting any very profound analysis, I am merely proposing to lay out in orderly fashion a number of commonplace notions, in the hope of tidying up some processes of ordinary thought. I call them commonplace, and so they are; but even the commonplace things are often overlooked or confused. It is precisely at the gaps in an articulated process that errors in reasoning creep in. I would hope also that this elementary stocktaking will do something for our vocabulary: not to introduce learned terms, but to realize that quite ordinary everyday words can, and should, be used with precision. Readers may care to try their hands at explaining the differences between such sets of words as *uninterested* and *disinterested; sensual* and *sensuous,* and *sensate* and *sentient; imply* and *infer; meticulous* and *punctilious; small* and *little; surprise* and *astonish; expect* and *anticipate; grey* and *gray;* and then to compare their answers with those of colleagues and with the reference dictionaries. The results may prove unexpected, even shocking. For in uncultivated speech, such words are used with disheartening coarseness, and many would treat the words within each set as interchangeable.

STEPS IN THE DEVELOPMENT OF AN IDEA

In table 9.1 I have a brief sketch of the main levels and means of reflection by which scientific ideas of a certain class evolve. I shall confine my remarks to the experiences of alert minds engaged in scientific thought.

Unprocessed Experiences

The process by which perceptions were first separated from passive sensory bombardment is lost in evolutionary history. There

Table 9.1. Steps in the Development of an Idea

Domain of Enquiry	Method	Illustration
Unprocessed experiences	Casual observation	There is much nucleic acid in every cell.
Data	Directed enquiry (discernment)	There are four nucleotides in nucleic acid, adenosine (A), cytosine (C), guanine (G), and either thymidine (T) (in DNA) or Uracil (U) (in RNA).
Facts	Analysis	The molar ratio of A to T is close to unity and so is that of G to C (Chargaff's law).
Ideas	Surmise	Nucleic acid consists of two matching (complementary) strands, each C being paired with a G and each A with a T or a U (the Watson-Crick model).
Insight	Illation (or unprecedented conjecture)	Nucleic acid represents a degenerate, punctuated, triplet code for the building of the protein molecule, one amino acid at a time.

is no such thing as a virgin intellect. Our first conscious contacts are typically with almost unprocessed experiences: when an artist recaptures this primordial state of pure wonder, he is hailed as a great genius. Medical students who know nothing of wardcraft will nonetheless automatically start to note the ways and the degrees in which people differ. In this they are retracing the steps of the early physicians, poets, novelists (many of them physicians), playwrights, painters, and all the rest. This experience is universal; yet the physician, however sophisticated or experienced, should never lose touch with it. It is only too easy to fall so in love with decorous abstractions as to leave earthy reality behind. That course makes for both bad science and bad medicine. Even if the common touch is to be preserved as nothing more than an idiom in which to communicate with the patient, it is still important; for most patients do not live in a world of abstractions, and their concern with concrete reality is increased when they are worried or in pain.

It is amazing how often clinicians, for lack of explicit fact, have to fall back on common experiences that they have picked up quite casually in clinical practice. Much of it would not stand any close scientific scrutiny and finds no description in the textbooks. Those looking for a simple research topic can usually quarry some valuable nuggets by studying "what everybody knows." Surprisingly often, what everybody knows turns out to be inaccurate in detail.

There is a contrasting aspect: all the things that the physician never notices.

Example 9.1. According to the textbooks (67), in the Marfan syndrome the palate has an unusual shape; but since physicians rarely look at the palate unless they expect to find an abnormality, they personally may have little to interpret their findings against.

Data

Once we start to pick and choose the things to which we will pay attention, we are no longer dealing in simple experiences, but in data. It is a mistake to imagine either that data fall into our laps or that data form a completely unprejudiced basis for enquiry. At this stage we have already started editing our experiences, and dismissing some features as noise, as distraction. If a patient were to say that he had lost his appetite because he had been cursed by a gypsy, most physicians would not even record the fact; psychiatrists would perhaps infer that the patient is superstitious or suggestible; but none would treat the fact of the event as important in its own right. I do not imply that their attitude is at all incorrect. Nevertheless, it is an attitude, which is separate from the unprocessed information itself, and which is used to edit the information. At a less trivial level, the whole of the process of clinical examination is conducted with discernment.

Example 9.2. In neurological diseases, the pupils and their reactions are of cardinal importance, eye color (except for albinism) of almost no interest.

Example 9.3. Physical examination by percussion is often of major value in the lungs; in the heart, rarely and little; in the thigh, never and none.

Example 9.4. In obtaining a random sample from the population, the type and scope of sampling (whether representative, probabilistic, stratified) is of major importance. If it is ideally performed, however, *the order in which the subjects are recruited* contains no information about the population. (In actual practice, it may bear on the quality of the observations and trends in the observer's acumen, which is likely to be influenced by accumulated interest and by boredom.)

Facts

While the data are chosen with clear objectives in mind, they will not in general be twenty-four-carat gold. Their meaning may be hidden by various contaminants that we shall discuss in some detail later. As we saw in chapter 7, there are *errors of measurement* that may be purely technical, or due to the inner nature of what is being observed (for instance, the indefiniteness of an end point or the randomness of radioactive decay). There may be *systematic variation* that may, or may not, have been recognized. There is, for instance, a seasonal variation in the level of cholesterol in blood; a variation of body temperature with the menstrual cycle; a diurnal variation in the secretion of growth hormone. Height is related to age. There may be *confounding of effects*, such as we discussed in chapter 3.

Example 9.5. Patients have more atherosclerosis with age; but as a cause of heart disease, this disorder is mixed up with many other changes (in weight, amount of exercise taken, responsibilities, income, experience, etc.) that also occur with age. The effects of these factors may be difficult to disentangle from the effects of atherosclerosis.

To arrive at facts (that is, ideally, true statements about authentic entities, their properties, how they relate to one another, and so forth) may thus demand careful analysis and unusual intellectual penetration. Again, we may deplore the naive confusion between facts and either data or experiences. Facts are conclusions from data, by a process of reasoning, in accordance with prescribed principles of inference. They thus depend on both data (which demand directed enquiry) and processing (which involves conventions of analysis).

Sometimes the facts are taken in at a glance, as in the gestalt (or informal pattern recognition). What a radiologist learns from a cardiac silhouette or a dysmorphologist does from a face are often facts of this type. It is remarkable the speed with which the experienced practitioner will go through what, expounded in detail, proves to be a most complicated piece of reasoning. Often, when challenged, even he may have difficulty in reconstructing it. In such cases there is some risk of confusing data with facts, confusion which may give rise to more or less serious errors. What is more, people skilled at such arts are often impatient about distinguishing between data and the inference (just as some are impatient about the distinction between symptoms and signs). It is when one tries to write a computer program to distill fact from data that the subtlety of the reasoning and the need for explicit criteria become apparent.

Yet the subconscious clinical inference may be in error.

Example 9.6. Consider the patient with left-sided abdominal pain and tenderness. The clinician, without recognizing any process of inference at all, excludes appendicitis. It may be only at laparotomy that he realizes that the patient has appendicitis with complete transposition of the viscera. One would be foolish to dismiss this error because it is rare. It is precisely because it is rare that the mistake is apt to happen; and the aggregate of such *kinds* of rare oversights may amount to a formidable amount of error (just as the aggregate of thousands of rare genetic disorders amounts to a large proportion of clinical disease). One does well to remember also that however rare the mistake, it happens in 100 percent of the patient concerned.

Sometimes the process of reasoning is highly explicit and intricate. In bedside Medicine, elaborate inference is well illustrated by the neurological diagnosis. For since the brain is inaccessible to the ordinary means of physical examination, diagnosis must depend on inferences from indirect signs. Since the operation of a hierarchy of mechanisms at various levels of complexity is being expressed through (in Sherrington's telling phase) a final common path, the arguments may be extremely subtle and the findings often ambiguous. Neurological disorders of speech and of bladder control are notorious examples.

Simple inspection of the laboratory results may be of little help; and an adequate analysis of the raw data may be dauntingly intricate. One may cite as examples electroencephalography, the dynamics of blood platelets, and the most spectacular example of all, computerized axial tomography (CAT scanning). For all of them, the analysis demands not only a computer but a command of some rather formidable mathematics. In such cases, there is relatively little risk of confusing data with the results from these extremely elaborate processes of inference.

Ideas

For the most part, the foregoing are technical procedures, that is, they consist of the application of an agreed theory, by standardized methods, to stereotyped data. CAT scanning, for example, is a quite remarkable advance in clinical science, duly acknowledged by the award of a Nobel prize. But the practising radiologist does not need to be competent in the underlying theory; the calculations are left to a computer program.

There are many instances, however, in which a fundamental problem is *to devise* the refined theory or method for analyzing some more or less well-defined problem.

Example 9.7. Echocardiography, a special case of sonography, was a technical development of the method of percussion long used by the clinician. Because the frequency of the ultrasound used is much higher, and the speed of interpretation (being visual) is much faster, it has higher resolving power both in space and in time. Thus, not only can one examine small structures, such as the cusps of a valve, one can also study almost continuously how they move. The surgeon, following the course of paralytic ileus by percussing the abdomen from hour to hour, is using the same process as the cardiologist examining the mitral valve by echocardiography; but he is doing so on a scale that is many orders of magnitude coarser both in space and in time. However, even the much older bedside percussion is a technique that its author, Laennec, learnt from his father's wine trade (rapping a barrel being one of the ways of deciding how full it is); and that in turn may have been borrowed from the way in which a blind man finds his way by listening to the echoes from the tapping of his stick.

When I call their current use "technical," I am not belittling the developments of these refinements as intellectual feats. Moreover, in many cases not only were technical solutions demanding but, at the outset, there was no assurance of success. The failures in such attempts are most likely, or at least most readily apparent, where some major theoretical development is involved that furnishes a criterion for measuring success.

Example 9.8. The development of the first method for studying blood flow to the brain in man (68) involved an analogue of the method of measuring blood flow to the kidney (11). But the logic is more intricate, and the data must be collected and timed with far greater precision. Also, since particular facts could not be obtained about the cerebral circulation, flow had to be expressed per unit of brain mass rather than in absolute terms. Moreover, the logic depends on certain assumptions about connections among the branches of the main arteries to the brain. Any, or all, of these aspects might have undermined the method. The theoretical arguments furnished a way of exposing the defects in the method if they had indeed been of unacceptable magnitude. The method triumphantly passed the test. With modern developments, there are now more sensitive ways of detecting inadequacies in a particular set of studies of cerebral blood flow than in one of renal blood flow.

But not all such endeavors lead to successful refinement.

Example 9.9. The crippling technical problems of assaying the blood level of the enzyme creatine phosphokinase (which, reason suggests, should be high in diseases in which muscles waste) has been a thorn in the side of the geneticist for many years (69).

Insight

At times, further advance in a field is possible only by an adventurous, but prudent, foray into the unknown. A distinguished his-

torian of science, Kuhn, has termed these steps "scientific revolutions" in a classical book (70). He contrasts them with the orderly
application of orthodox ideas to special topics, which he terms
"normal science." Kuhn seems to reserve the idea of scientific revolutions for rare, epochal, and rather disruptive ideas, such as Newton's gravitation or Einstein's relativity. He seems to set much store
by the *magnitude* of the change and its effects. He invented the
notion and is certainly entitled to use it as he sees fit. But much the
same kind of process is at work more or less continuously, the
distinguishing character (as I see it) being not so much its magnitude, its disruptiveness, or the extent of its impact as that it involves
jumping to some extent outside the entrenched principles of
inference.

Example 9.10. For the most part, the discovery and analysis of a
new variant of hemoglobin is now little more than a technical exercise in primary sequencing of a protein, which falls well within
orthodox biochemistry. But the notion that this protein has indeed
a highly patterned structure is due to the insight of Pauling and
Corey. Earlier it had been thought that a protein is a formless
colloid; and the discovery that it does have a detailed structure and
the identification of the kinds of components it may have (the
alpha helix, the beta pleated sheet) received a major impetus from
the remarkable series of frankly speculative papers by Pauling and
Corey (71), which went far beyond empirical experience, let alone
orthodoxy.

Because Kuhn's scale of reckoning does not seem to accommodate these smaller, but distinctive, contributions, we have applied
to this process of surmisal that goes beyond precedent the term
illation (72). Illation is an activity that attracts a miscellaneous group
of investigators. Dabblers in popular history tend to regard most
illative activities as rash, even insane; they take the rather pusillanimous attitude that those whose ideas pan out are geniuses and the
rest are fools. They must be embarrassed by those scholars typified
by Descartes, who is a genius because his coordinate geometry
works, and a fool because his cosmology of vortices does not. In our
own time we have seen reaction to the theory of continental drift
change from its being seen as the absurd obsession of a crank to its
being considered the spectacular insight of genius. One could go
through the writings of Virchow, the patriarch of tissue pathology,
and find pages of "profound contributions" interspersed with
pages of "arrant nonsense." (I quote the considered judgment of a
discerning colleague.) One is apt to forget that both are the product of the one person. A sensible assessment is that whoever takes

intellectual risks is going to make some mistakes and that those who take no risks, even in private, may extend knowledge but will never advance insight. But woe betide those that are adventurous to no purpose!

PROPHETIC THEORIES

Particularly in biology, there is a widespread arrogance of the practical that (despite the Pauling-Corey theory, just stated) claims that theoretical biology has no useful separate existence. The hostile grudgingly admit that theorists help now and again to clean up their own data for them but they claim that they never open up entirely new fields of enquiry of their own. This image is quite false of other sciences, notably the most respected of all, physics; and in living off imported methods, the practical are (often unwittingly) demolishing their own thesis.

Example 9.11. X-ray crystallography, the cornerstone of most of our knowledge about the tertiary structure of protein, is critically dependent on Fourier analysis. But Fourier did not devise his theory to meet the needs of protein chemists. He was pursuing a line of abstract enquiry into the mathematical theory of numerical analysis many years before X-ray crystallography.

Example 9.12. What fragments we have about the precise formal analysis of homeostasis have descended through the cybernetics of Norbert Wiener (73) from two hundred years of theoretical development of differential equations and functional analysis.

Example 9.13. Aphasia would have been a much more confused field were it not for the insights furnished by linguistic theory.

Example 9.14. The showpiece of genetics, Mendel's classical experiments, illustrates the point nicely. Its germinal role in biology is beyond debate. But the common image portrays him as a benign, uncomplicated monk with sharp observation doing simple herbal studies in a monastery garden and arriving at conclusions that compelled him by their very simplicity. Nothing could be farther from the facts. Far from being a simple gardener, Mendel studied mathematics for three years at the University of Vienna and was an accredited teacher of mathematics. There is evidence that far from being inspired by empirical studies, Mendel was trying out a preconceived idea*. Indeed, Fisher (33) was critical because Mendel's

---

*A recent paper (Soudek D. "Gregor Mendel and the people around him [commemorative of the centennial of Mendel's death]." *Amer J Hum Genet*, 36:295–99, 1984) makes illuminating reading.

data fitted the prediction of his model suspiciously well; and Dunn (74), himself a distinguished geneticist, suggested that Mendel's experiments on peas led not so much to the discovery as to the demonstration of his laws. Far from being at once welcomed with open arms by the practical biologists, Mendel's discoveries were, and remained for forty years, utterly beyond their grasp, perhaps because they deal with abstract ideas rather than with matters that could be seen with the naked eye. It has been suggested to me by Dr. V. A. McKusick that it was Flemming's histological discovery of the chromosomes that (by furnishing a "local habitation" for the gene) rescued Mendelism from exile. Its neglect remains one of the most remarkable examples of obtuseness in the history of practical science. As Fisher pointed out (75), Mendelism was the very model needed to release Darwinism from a stalemate in its attempts to account for conservation of genetically beneficial traits that tended to be spared by selection.

Illative genius lies in discerning how far it is profitable to go, with a reasonable chance of useful discovery, beyond orthodox thought, and (as a safeguard against error) to know at every step what has been proved and how well; what part is questionable; and what part is pure surmise. This critical judgment is necessary for all who read medical literature. Even the most august journals publish much that is specious, and most claims will be discredited sooner or later. Enthusiasms keep the interest alive; but the solid beliefs of the responsible scientist or clinician have a long half-life and do not bob up and down like corks on the sea of fashionable conjecture. Kuhn's perception is sound that normal science is important as well as scientific revolution.

AN ILLUSTRATION

The foregoing scheme must not be seen as a piece of rigid scaffolding. All useful research partakes of each of the above steps; the greatest inspirations may be in the first step (Smithies discovered starch gel electrophoresis by noticing how washing blue behaves in domestic starch) or in the last (Kekulé conceived the spatial structure that accounted for the remarkable stability of the benzene ring in the course of a dream).

Example 9.15. The top illustration given in the last column of table 9.1 must be taken in relative terms. When I class the ubiquity of nucleic acid in cells as "casual observation," I obviously do not mean that anybody without skilled biochemistry would even be aware of it. But it is casual in the sense that it was found simply by routine chemical analysis; nucleic acid was analyzed because it was there, not because anybody had been specifically looking for it. Even so, forty years ago its function was unknown. Systematic study showed its components; and Chargaff (76) discovered the law of the quantitative relationship between the pairs of nucleotides. The next step—the Watson-Crick model (77)—seems in hindsight an obvious one, although filling in the technical details and confirming them were by no means trivial. That it was a profound perception is shown by the fact that although Chargaff was trembling on the brink of this discovery, he did not, in fact, make it. But this step illustrates nicely the emergence, from a law that can be merely stated, of insight that can be grasped. In the same fashion, Kepler had shown three regular laws of planetary motion: their elliptical paths; the relationship of distance to periodicity; and the constancy of the "area swept out" in unit time. But Chargaff's law and Kepler's laws, despite their generality, *might* have been coincidences or approximations*; it is a bold scientist who would pronounce them universally and exactly true. Watson and Crick's helix and Newton's gravitation put forward in each case a single idea, at once easy to grasp and economical in structure, that explained a set of laws, well substantiated but conceptually unmotivated; and both then led on to various verifiable predictions, many of which were not readily deduced from the original set of laws. (The behavior of the classical "three-body" system of astrophysics is a famous instance. It can be readily, if somewhat untidily, solved by numerical means, on Newton's principle. It would have been a formidable undertaking to approach it from Kepler's laws.)

The fifth item in table 9.1, insight, is the most subtle one to analyze. It involves the idea that each combination of three of the nucleotides (A, C, G, T, U) given in table 9.1 is a code unit for one amino acid. It is illative in various ways, of which the most important is that it is without precedent. Nobody before (to my knowledge) had ever shown in nature the existence of a physiological code, a code in the technical sense that the message bears a purely arbitrary relationship to the operation.

Example 9.16. What does CAU mean? Viewed in one way it is, as it were, a linguistic codeword meaning "falls."† The same letters in the genetic code mean *histidine*. But the arbitrariness of the code in

---

*For instance, at the time of this writing, it is unclear whether Bode's law (which deals with the relationship between the sizes and positions of the planets in the solar system, see Murphy [12]) really is a scientific law and not merely a mnemonic device.

†In Catalan.

both instances is shown by the fact that histidine and falling have nothing to do with each other.

To take this step of invoking a code was a bold one. It makes an appeal to Occam's principle of economy: that the coding unit must be as short as possible.* Each nucleotide (either in DNA or in RNA) allows four choices, so that a code word n units in length would allow 4^n combinations. The number of known amino acids to be coded for is greater than 4^2 (or 16) and less than 4^3 (or 64), and hence the code word must have at least three units and need have no more. Even so, 64 words is too many; either some are not used, or there are multiple code words with the same meaning (a feature called "degeneracy" of the code, a metaphor borrowed from the theory of differential equations). The actual code proves to be degenerate and in a surprisingly uneven way. There are six words for leucine, only one for methionine. (The analogy with ordinary language is intriguing.) It is not at all clear to me how far the nature and extent of this degeneracy is determined. I have said that the code is arbitrarily, and not logically, related to the amino acid; but if we knew enough about the evolution† of the code, that claim might not be at all true. Analogously, students of etymology and linguistics have by no means despaired of relating the form of language to its meaning. To set up a simple dichotomy that either the code determines the pattern of selection or selection determines the pattern of the code is shallow.

THE USES OF IDEAS IN MEDICINE

There is a vast literature on the history of ideas, which is a matter best handled by the historians and others competent in this field. I will undertake a humbler and more practical task. Why do we need ideas in medicine? Why do we need anything more than the facts?

Compactness

The first and most obvious answer is that not only are books and computers much more capacious, efficient, and accurate repositories of fact than the human mind is, they allow increasingly more rapid means of recall. If there were nothing more to Medicine than

*One factor favoring a short code unit is the tolerable mutation rate, which will depend on the number of nucleotides.

†A colleague has pointed out to me that there has been a considerable body of speculative literature on this topic.

access to fact, vastly more of the medical curriculum should be devoted to learning to use computers, and it would be quite useless to memorize anything. Now I am sure that nobody believes that way of putting it to be a fair representation of Medicine. Those who do not understand academic and professional skill have a crass preoccupation with fact: they suppose that lawyers memorize the statutes, physicians learn lists of symptoms and signs, engineers learn logarithms. A sage, they fancy, is someone with a prodigious memory, and a mathematician knows every formula in existence. Certainly one can set too little store by fact. But the scholar is distinguished less by how much he has learned than by *what* he has chosen to learn and how he makes use of what he knows.

Example 9.17. The idea that a change in the structure of hemoglobin would lead to disordered functioning and perhaps disease might have occurred to anybody. It was first demonstrated in sickle hemoglobin as an incidental, even an accidental, by-product of Ingram's work on "fingerprinting" hemoglobin (54). This discovery started a fashion; and while in the early stages the fact mongers could keep track of all hemoglobins, Dr. V. A. McKusick informs me that at the time of this writing there are 556 different hemoglobins recorded. But 556 facts or 556 specimens do not mean 556 ideas. A hematology text with even ten lines on each would make monstrously dull reading, a prospect that would get gloomier with each new edition.

It seems obvious that as a countercurrent to steady multiplication of fact, there must be a steady process of conflation or unification. Even an obsessive hematologist cannot reasonably or usefully memorize the details: the best repository for them is McKusick's catalogue (14) or a computer. Both the scholar and the clinician will try to find some new way of looking at the entire subject. One may identify the topic, not as a study of every individual hemoglobin, but as one of physiological *dimensions*. For instance, various hemoglobins may lead to any of the following patterns.

1. They may take up too little oxygen and cause *cyanosis* (the methemoglobins).
2. They may have such avidity for oxygen that it is only by an increased mass of red cells (*polycythemia*) that what oxygen they do release will be sufficient for the tissues (the high-affinity hemoglobins).
3. They may be easily destroyed, so that the red cells have a short *survival* and the patient suffers permanently from a hemolytic anemia (unstable hemoglobins).

4. They may assume abnormal forms, so that the red cells have a bizarre *shape* under special circumstances (such as forms shaped like sickles when the oxygen level is low).
5. They may occur in the beta chains, so that they will have little impact until *after birth* (such as hemoglobins S and C).
6. They may be associated with *anemia* due to deficient production of hemoglobin (the thalassemias).

The list of characteristics could be extended, but not so fast as the list of individual hemoglobins. The point is that the clinical (as distinct from the genetic or evolutionary) implications lie, not in the identity of the hemoglobin, but in how it behaves. We could, of course, deal with hemoglobins in groups, that is, by classifying them. But there would probably be much more practical interest in knowing such specifications of a particular hemoglobin. One has thus replaced a list that is unlimited and already long, with a compact set of *dimensions of performance*. (This topic of dimensionality and cardinality will be resumed in chapter 12.)

Comprehension

A great part of creative thought seems to be the capacity to see new relationships among separate things. To see such relationships, one must be able to keep the several things in mind at once. The word *comprehension* is a particular evocative metaphor: it means that what one is thinking of is compact enough to be *grasped*.

However, this comprehensiveness is a property of ideas, not of words. Anybody who studies Medicine for long will see a tendency for the shallow to overload an idea that they do not understand with problems that they have not defined. Much the same set of unexplained diseases have at one time or another (depending on fashion) been ascribed to deficiency of a hypothetical vitamin, an unidentified virus, genetic factors with bizarre properties, autoimmune disease, stress, "the glands," focal sepsis, allergy, and the rest. The common effect has been, through overuse, to bring into disrepute ideas each of which has a sound, but limited, area of application. It is not enough that an idea should simplify; it must do it constructively.

But while simplicity guarantees nothing, one is wise to mistrust complexity. It is a sound rule that the longer the name given a disease, the less we know about it. Often the name is a lamentation over our difficulties, translated into a garbled version of a dead language; dead but, unfortunately, not forgotten. Any disease with a name of more than fifteen letters is almost certainly living beyond its intellectual means. Those who like mumbo jumbo (most of the laity and too many in the medical profession) are apt to despise words like *the gout* or *the cold* or *drunk* or *mad* or even *dead*. Surely, they suppose, doctors have not studied medicine for years, or patients paid their honest money, for answers in such simple terms! But their hearts are gladdened by diagnoses such as "agnogenic myeloid metaplasia" or "pseudoachondroplastic spondyloepiphyseal dysplasia" or "pityriasis lichenoides et varioliformis acuta," which tell us practically nothing about the disease.

On the principle that the more compact, the more comprehensible, and the greater the hope of insight, we must deplore any long word that adds neither precision nor understanding to a short one. I would tolerate *avitaminosis C* in place of the now rather quaint term *scurvy* and *streptococcal tonsillitis* for *sore throat* (provided that it is indeed in the tonsil and the cause is the streptococcus). But I can think of no circumstances in which good comes of saying *diaphorese* for *sweat;* or *visualize* for *see;* or *male sibling* for *brother*. The reader must not, of course, suppose that I am fanatically opposed to all technical words, even obscure ones. But I must have value for my money.

Example 9.18. The word *distichiasis* denotes that state in which *the roots of the eyelashes, instead of lying in a single row, lie in two parallel rows*. Although obscure, this term not only saves the long phrase in italics in the last sentence but denotes a sign in several genetic syndromes that at least furnishes information on the risk of transmission and helps in assessing the significance of other, somewhat puzzling, clinical findings.

Toughness

An idea must have a quality that I shall call toughness. It represents a sound compromise between two extreme states.

Rigidity. An idea is rarely the better for being totally rigid. Rigidity makes for a firm theory and for no-nonsense inference and prediction. It has all the admirable qualities of dogma (in the proper sense of that much-abused word): precision, compactness, freedom from ambiguity. Properly used, it does not substitute authority for truth. If it is true it is verifiable. If it is false, it is readily demolished. It does not, like the nondogmatic utterance, take a long time to die. The Watson-Crick model is dogmatic. It has nothing to offer in the way of intellectual calisthenics. Those who make deductions from it either understand it and prosper or do not and make fools of themselves. Such a state is sufficiently definite to be disputed and to be disproved, if false. In the hands of the theorist, at least, rigid models are apt to prove brittle. If the facts do not agree with the idea, the only alternative to discarding the facts is to bend the idea; and if the idea will not bend, it will break. If the model is almost right, but not quite, this outcome is a destructive one. Many universal statements are in peril. It is common wisdom that in Medicine one should avoid the terms *never* or *always*. Ideas that are always true usually turn out to be saying nothing at all.

Example 9.19. The idea that all people over seventy are senile is warranted if, and only if, we define *senile* as meaning over seventy. The statement thus reduces to the form "all people over seventy are over seventy." Empty, but quite safe.

The reader should be on the alert for statements of this kind (known as *tautologies*), which are definitions and nothing more, but often so disguised as to appear to be useful propositions. Of course, definitions, though always tautologous, have their uses; but they are not themselves facts or suitable topics for *scientific enquiry*. There is no point whatsoever in doing empirical studies on how many legs a quadruped has or in trying to find what proportion of patients have a level of blood cholesterol that falls in the top 10 percent.

Laxity. On the other hand an idea may be so shapeless that it would accommodate itself to any state of nature whatsoever. Trying to break the back of a jellyfish is a lost cause.

Evidential Merit

It is the custom to demand of what purports to be a scientific statement that it be *falsifiable,* that is, that there exist means by which it can be shown to be false if it is false. This leads to the empiric principle of falsifiability:

• *A scientific statement may be asserted to be true insofar as it could conceivably be shown to be false, if false.*

Scientists, speaking as scientists, cannot usefully say that there exist beings in the world that they cannot perceive; for if they cannot perceive them, then they cannot distinguish between the state in which they exist and the state in which they do not exist. (That evident fact, I am afraid, does not stop many from invoking science to bolster up such statements.)

Although it is a good watchdog, one must be careful not to abuse this principle of falsifiability, at least as it is usefully applied in Medicine.

What We Cannot Perceive Changes with Time. The claim that X-rays exist is falsifiable now, whereas it would have been neither verifiable nor falsifiable in the eighteenth century (always assuming that somebody had raised the question of their existence at that time). Claims that an idea is permanently nonfalsifiable cannot be scientific. They are warranted only if it can be shown that a statement is of its very nature nonfalsifiable: that is, if saying that the idea is falsifiable would lead to a contradiction.

Denials Also Are Propositions. Only some things that are not (by this criterion) true are therefore false. To say that something is false is also an assertion. Scientists require a reciprocal principle of authenticity.

• *A statement may be asserted to be false only insofar as it may conceivably be shown to be true, if true.*

If in the nature of things there is no way of proving something true, then the scientist may or may not believe it as he chooses. But, in my viewpoint, he is not entitled to a scientific statement that it is false.

Example 9.20. In an experiment designed to exclude all means of observation, one cannot assert, after the event, what happened. One cannot verify whether the laws of physics operate under conditions in which there are no observers or observing devices. In the clinical context, there is no possible way of determining what is going on in a completely undisturbed mind or body.

Some hold that the cutting edge of science consists of rejecting hypotheses: that data that repeatedly confirm the current theory soon lose what merit they have, and that real advances in science come from finding discrepancies between the data and the existing theory, which drive us to seek a deeper and more enriching theory. I have no doubt that there is merit in this view, especially in such fields as physics, where the theories are already clear, the data are transparent, and the besetting temptation is intellectual smugness. (I do not say that smugness is in the least common among physicists: merely that it may result, and it is all the more to be feared and the more devastating when it happens.) Rigor is an enviable quality, but not rigor mortis.

However I have misgivings about applying this principle to biology. While cold baths may be invigorating for the healthy, they may be lethal to the sick. So much of the concern in biology lies in trying to get started any heuristic theory whatsoever, however rough, that our surmises must be treated with some indulgence. Otherwise, scientists will become nihilistic about all theories and fall back into a mindless Baconian collection of facts. Though the principle must be applied with some caution, it is better to have a rough theory, even though its inadequacies are at once obvious, than to have a completely shapeless vision of the problem.

Example 9.21. The current stance of biologists is opposed to the view that evolution is a process with a purpose. In this view, to say that homeostatic mechanisms developed *in order to* maintain the inner environment is ruled out of court. The evolutionist would recast this notion in terms of what states are at a selective advantage. Nevertheless, by supposing that there is purpose, even without the necessary hard facts one can make a fairly good guess at how the body would respond if (say) the level of blood sugar were to become too low. And it is clear that the notion of purpose is not merely a mnemonic device (such as we use to remember the names of the cranial nerves).

Thus, one can make a case for the provisional usefulness of half-true theories. However, the least sign of smugness on the part of the biologist, any hint that he is resting on his (or more often other people's) laurels should call down the axe of criticism with a vengeance.

Not All Knowledge Is Empirical. Readers may protest that there are ways of arriving at truth other than empirical observation. Quite so. But then (tautologously) they are not empirical proofs; and insofar as the touchstone of scientific proof is *what happens,* empiricism falters where we cannot find out what happens.*

Proprositions May Be Undecidable. From the foregoing arguments, it follows that empirically at least, many statements may not legitimately be asserted to be either true or false.

The toughness that I am asking of a sound idea is a happy compromise between rigidity and spinelessness. It should be pliable, but not helpless. If it is pliable and not quite right, there is some prospect that we may be able to modify the form of the idea without doing ultimate violence to it.

PROBLEMS

9.1. Analyze the pairs of italicized words on the first page of this chapter, and then compare your conclusions with those in detailed dictionaries.

9.2. The diagram shown in figure 9.1 is made up by starting from the central square and by adding further generations of

---

*I personally believe many things that are outside the domain of empirical science: I would mention free will, responsibility and imputability, beauty, truth, inspiration, and deeper matters still—all beyond the scope and methods of this book.

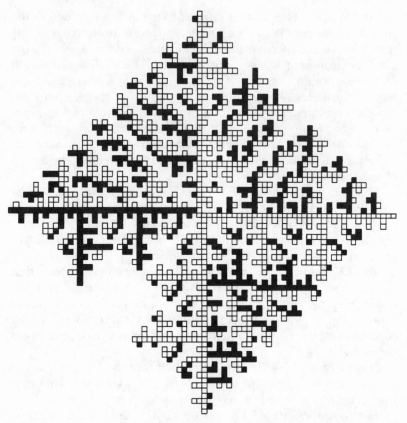

Figure 9.1. The diagram shown starts as a white square in the very center of the diagram and grows out from it. The problem is to discern the pattern of growth, including deciding whether it involves any random component.

squares in accordance with a set of rules. The first forty generations have been completed. See if you can find a principle of symmetry. Would you say that this is a deterministic process or is there a random element involved? What would you imagine the rules are?

9.3. Translate the following flowers of rhetoric into brief, sensible, and useful English: upper and lower extremities; careful physical examination revealed that; paroxysmal nocturnal dyspnea; no organomegaly was present; singultus; family history was noncontributory; bilaterally symmetrical on both sides. (This last blossom comes from the most distinguished contemporary textbook of medicine.)

9.4. Analyze and compare the following statements.

a. It is better to have a normal prostate with a high acid phosphatase level than a cancerous prostate with a low level.

b. It is better to be obese without being overweight than thin and overweight.

c. "For such a stupid man he is remarkably intelligent."

d. It is better to be a carrier of hemophilia with a high factor VIII level than not to be a carrier and have a low level.

e. After adjustments have been made for differences in mortality rate at different ages, all human beings have the same life span.

f. "I don't know what my mother died of, but it was not anything serious."

9.5. Write a step-by-step recipe for
a. Constructing a diagram of the outline of a crescent moon
b. Arranging ten unequal numbers in increasing order of magnitude
c. Plaiting three strands of rope.

9.6. Identify which of the following statements are verifiable, falsifiable, or neither.
a. During undisturbed sleep, human beings do not dream.
b. Penicillin has cured the common cold in a particular person.
c. The skin lesions in pityriasis rosea never itch.
d. Two minds cannot occupy the same physical space simultaneously.
e. On average, body weight is reduced by pheochromocytoma.
f. The height in a person at the fiftieth percentile is less than average.
g. All statements that are not true are false.

10 | Measures

Since the perceptions of Galileo, we have come to think that the things of the physical world can be put in three sufficient terms: time, mass, and length. We now call it the CGS (centimeter-gram-second) system. To have founded this system of cardinal dimensions is a remarkable feat. It is so widely used and (in physics) so rarely found wanting, that we hardly grasp its importance. We may think it a logical necessity such as must be obvious to everybody.

Yet it is clear that this science cannot easily cater to other fields such as biology and, for all I know to the contrary, cannot cater to them at all. Nevertheless, biologists may wish to deal with their evidence in quantitative terms. The reasons for doing so are many. Scholars are right to be concerned about the observer bias that might occur if their answers were nothing better than judgments that are not subject to scrutiny. Where chance plays a large part, they will have to use quantitative analysis to take due account of it. The biologist may wish to measure how alike relatives are as a gauge of how important genetic factors are. The pharmacologist needs to compare how well two drugs work. Some of these problems can be dealt with by counting categorical outcomes rather than by measuring quantities. Patients either die or get better; they are male or female; they have, or do not have, such and such a blood group; and so forth. However, these methods often lack statistical power and refinement; and they are by no means without problems of their own, as we shall see presently.

If measurements are to be used—as when the geneticist turns from the categorical methods of Mendel to the quantitative methods of Galton and Fisher, or the physician turns from the nominal diagnosis of the gout to interpreting the concentration of uric acid—there is need for a scale of measurement. Sometimes the scale is natural and obvious.

Example 10.1. When Mendel looked at the genetics of height in pea plants, he found that they fall naturally into two kinds—short and tall—a grouping that was clear enough for his needs and did not call for any actual measurements. When Galton, unaware of Mendel's work, looked at height in man, he found quite a different story: no clear grouping, but a smooth gradation of size. To grapple with it formally, he had need of a measurement, and happily for him, height could be expressed as a simple value on the well-known scale of length.

Example 10.2. When Galton and the psychometrists came to do the same for intelligence, however, they got into rather deep waters. There are two main difficulties. On the one hand, it has never been claimed that intelligence has anything directly to do with length, mass, or time. Thus, it becomes necessary to make a quite new kind of scale on which intelligence could be measured, one, however, that will have properties that are unknown and not at all easy to guess. On the other hand, even when the scale has been chosen, the distribution of the results has been found, the reproducibility and other working properties of the system have been established, and even the parts that genetics and teaching have had in determining the trait of interest, we still have to ask ourselves what the outcomes mean.

Example 10.3. I do not think that any psychologist would now wish to make any claims that handedness is a sign of low intelligence or is a disease in itself. Yet purely for the sake of argument, let us examine the question. If it is found empirically that the left-handed are in all other ways as bright as the right-handed, then it seems that handedness does not tell us anything about intelligence. If we found that left-handed people are duller, then there is some chance that the fact that they are dull will be used to prop up the idea that left-handedness is evidence of mental dulness. If the belief that handedness is a significant measure of intelligence is founded on the agreement between it and (say) the ability to use analogies or to repeat numbers backwards, then there is no need to test for handedness. Because of how we have set up the rules of evidence, we may tell as much from the criteria by which dulness was validated in lefthanded people in the first place as we can from examining for handedness.

This argument applies to any new test whatsoever. If the new test agrees with other results from established tests, and does nothing else, it does not help; but if it does not agree, one interpretation would be that the new test is untrustworthy. On this argument, a new test is either superfluous or misleading. But that result prompts a criticism. How could we ever get started with the idea that a new sign throws any light on intelligence if it cannot be justified in itself and requires to be propped up by some other criteria? How is an attribute ever to be converted into a criterion?*

This line of thought paints a very gloomy picture of any scale of measurement that we make up; the reader might wonder whether it is ever possible to get any further in a field if a new test is to be dismissed unless it always leads to the same answer as older and better-known tests already in use (in which case the new test tells us nothing new). Before we try to find a more hopeful answer, it would be wise to see what there is to learn from example 10.3, which is typical of many.

Would we have been better off if we had a natural scale of intelligence given us without having to make one up? For the most part, perhaps, yes. But we must not overrate the usefulness of a natural measure just because it is there to use.

Example 10.4. In trying to compare how good several paintings are, we could find their widths or their areas; and I am sure that even a blind man could by touch alone tell big paintings from small. But while the measurement is exact enough, I do not myself think that it would tell us much about how good the painting is. However, we might argue in vain as to why it does not. Sound judges will no doubt agree fairly well about which are the better paintings. If their opinions are to be the bench mark (in effect, the *defining* criterion) of good painting, then it follows at once that no assessment can be better than these opinions. But how do we assure ourselves that the judges are sound? Clinical medicine is full of examples of diseases that physicians have tried to define by some measurement. Some succeed more than others; but the mere fact that something can be measured with great nicety is not the only, or even the main, warrant we should think about.

MEANING

It seems to me that one fundamental issue is meaning—the notion that beyond a measurement or, more generally, beyond the mere observation of the properties of things, there is something

---

*Yet nobody would deny that in fact at a critical point in 1959 the defining criterion of Down's syndrome changed from being a set of clinical findings to being a disorder in the number of chromosomes (78).

more fundamental with which we are ultimately concerned: that it is this fundamental thing that we are trying to find. The object of interest is not merely the manifestations, which are nothing more than the evidence that we have of its existence and quality. It has been fashionable, in the last half century or so, to decry this notion and to suggest that meaning is nothing but the signification of words. From the standpoint of medicine, one sees that this claim contains much truth. But some extremists have pushed the argument to such absurd extremes as to make one wonder whether their proponents have ever actually done any science or even watched a scientist at work. If they wish to outlaw the broader uses of *meaning*, they are free to do so. And so much the worse for their reputation for wisdom. We shall continue to find plenty of fruitful use in Medicine for these notions so patronizingly banished.

This discussion may sound exasperatingly abstract. Let me give a few examples that not only will make it more concrete but may persuade even the most practically minded reader that meaning is very much to the point. Let us start with a lay illustration.

Example 10.5. Let us try to imagine what it must have been like when untutored intelligences first looked at the moon. They saw it regularly going through a cycle of changes: first invisible; then crescentic, semicircular, gibbous, circular; then declining in the reverse order (fig. 10.1A). To the naked eye the shapes are smooth geometrical forms and nothing else. Moreover as it goes through this cycle the moon also changes its position in the sky. Then somebody took the imaginative step which may be represented by putting in the dotted lines in figure 10.1B, and grasped that the pattern is exactly what one would expect of a sphere perpetually lit on one face by the sun, and rotating about the earth. It led at once to the idea that the light is entirely reflected. Now at this stage, the perception has in no way added to the body of empirical evidence though it has worked wonders with its *evidentness*. It has rearranged the evidence long available to everybody so as to give it what (in defiance of the critics) we may call meaning. (It has nothing whatsoever to do with purely verbal meaning.) And the richness of this meaning carries its own conviction which has nothing whatsoever to do with proof either.

Now what do we mean by *meaning* in this example?

1. The image imparts coherence to what one has observed. It is much easier to remember the facts once one has grasped their meaning. In this, meaning is quite different from a purely mnemonic device. I can remember the function of the troch-

A

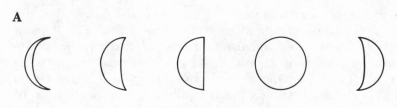

B

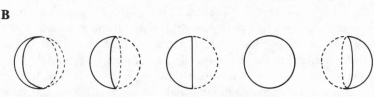

Figure 10.1. Meaning and illation. Diagram *A* represents the raw data of experience about the phases of the moon. Diagram *B* represents an illative interpretation in which the dashed lines indicate the surmised outline of those parts of the moon not lit by the sun and hence not seen. The persuasive character of this latter step comes, not from the addition of facts of proof or of formal inference, but from meaning.

lear nerve by knowing that it used to be called the *pathetic* nerve and that it makes the eye "look down and out." This last example is quite a different kind of aid to memory. It is merely an amusing pun, like Müller's mnemonic that the blood on the left side of the heart (like the politicians of the left) is red. The pattern of the moon's apparent changes in shape corresponds to something that we believe is actually happening, although it was not obvious until it was imagined. It is typical of this kind of advance that, once made, it seems trivial.

2. The perception leads to more detailed predictions that can be verified. One might not know the facts explicitly, but from this model it is at once obvious that when the moon is full, it will be at its zenith at midnight; that it is only then that it will ever be eclipsed by the earth, and so on.

3. The pattern forms a basis for generalization. If we saw another heavenly body that behaved in the same way, we would at once grasp what was happening.

4. In suitable cases, meaning provides a basis for rational action, where a limited experience may give us no sound empirical justification for it.

Now a theorist may argue that whoever made this surmise about the moon immediately put to the test the predictions included under point 2. Certainly that would be a professional scientist's response. But it would not be the response of the child; and I daresay, it was not the response of the primitive mind to whom it occurred. In both cases, even the insight of the illuminated sphere alone would carry major conviction.

Let us take a more specifically medical illustration.

Example 10.6. The posteroanterior X-ray of the chest in a patient with a pleural effusion typically shows that the fluid throws a crescentic shadow, the highest point being in the axilla (fig. 10.2A). Some twenty years before X-rays were discovered, a physician, Ellis, had reported (79) that in a pleural effusion the characteristic dulness to percussion is more marked in the axillary line. Apparently this sign had been noted by Damoiseau even earlier (80). Here are two facts nicely in agreement. Why should this uneven

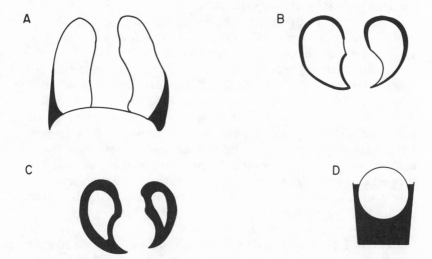

Figure 10.2. Meaning and illation. Radiological signs of pleural effusion and their origin. *A:* The curved black shadow in the axilla is characteristic. *B* and *C:* Sections through the upper and lower chest, showing the variable depth of fluid (in solid black) that X-rays must penetrate in a posterioanterior radiograph (that is, from above downwards in the two diagrams). Because the fluid collects under gravity at the lower part of the chest, the fluid is more abundant and the thickness less variable there. *D:* A mechanical model showing how the varying thickness of water, left when a balloon is put in a bucket of water, produces cusps at the sides. In the interest of simplicity, the sharpness of the limits of the balloon have been exaggerated. In reality, the edges would be much more diffuse (after Davis et al., 82).

distribution of the fluid happen? There was some informal speculation that as the fluid accumulates, it compresses the lung, and the latter collapses somewhat. It was supposed that the structure of the lung is such that the axillary part collapses more easily and sucks the fluid up nearby. This explanation can never have seemed very plausible, since the collapse of the lung was supposed to be a passive one due to compression by the fluid that is being accommodated. But it is not being sucked anywhere. Indeed, the theory is quite false. In 1935 Kaunitz (81) showed that if one puts into the pleura radio-opaque material of a density low enough to float to the top of the fluid, the upper limit of the fluid so defined does not curve upwards as the shadow of the fluid on the commonplace X-ray does, but is at the same level, back, front, and laterally. The fluid certainly tends to gravitate to the bottom of the pleural sack. The impression that it is concentrated in the axilla is an illusion due to the fact that the greatest thickness of fluid through which the X-rays pass lies in the axilla (fig. 10.2B and C) and the depth of the fluid *viewed end on* is much the same at all levels below the top. Variation in the *thickness* of fluid between the lung and the surface in the upper parts creates the illusion of uneven levels. When one grasps this explanation, it carries sudden and firm conviction. Davis and associates (82), who furnished this explanation, demonstrated the same effect by taking an X-ray of a bucket of water in which a balloon of air had been centrally placed (fig. 10.2D). But even without this evidence, their explanation would have carried complete conviction; and again the conviction is due, not to proof, but to *meaning* when it illuminated the same set of well-known facts suitably rearranged. Nevertheless, this triumphant explanation has created a new problem, for it does not explain why Damoiseau and Ellis had noticed the differences on percussion, a finding that could not have been an illusion prompted by the X-ray findings (which did not exist at the time).

Example 10.7. One could cite many instances from psychiatric practice of the diagnostic richness of meaning. Psychoanalytical methods of interpretation are at times abused; and weaker surmises do not persuade the critical mind. But among the masters, there are plenty of instances in which an assembly of apparently unrelated, and individually uninterpretable, facts suddenly all fall neatly into place when one perceives them from the right standpoint. Much the same is true of a set of neurological findings that one tries to account for by a single localized lesion.

The point I would stress is that, as science is commonly pictured by, and for, the laity, rather too much emphasis is put on proof at the expense of meaning. It is amusing to read the aphorisms of Sherlock Holmes, who had the oddest misconceptions as to how he solved his cases. Amongst other errors, he supposed that what he called on was proof, when most of his triumphs (including the strange case of the dog in the night, and the missing dumbbell) are exercises, not in proof or deduction at all, but in imaginatively finding, for some odd combination of facts, a surmise that he then proceeded to test. It is from meaning that the theory comes, and (a property we noted above) implicative meaning suggests how it might be confirmed.

The successful leap of imagination is often regarded as incapable of analysis, as a transcendent act of genius, beyond all comprehension. I, for one, do not find this idea plausible, helpful, or enlightening. One might compare it with an admirable (and easily understood) account by Polya, a distinguished mathematician, of how one can go about solving a new type of mathematical problem (83). One feature of this process, for instance, is a proper use of intellectual freedom: the idea that something one glibly regards as fixed and rigid, something not to be questioned, may after all not be quite so unyielding. Of course it would be foolhardy to kick over the traces altogether; but one may find that a little slack may be cautiously introduced with little harm and much benefit.

Example 10.8. There was a stage in the history of mathematics at which it was easy to see what 10^1, 10^2, and 10^3 meant: the first, a line of length ten units; the second, a square of side ten units; the third, a cube of side ten units. When Napier had the courage to imagine other states, such as 10^4 or $10^{2.5}$ or $10^{-2.7}$, none of which has any obvious geometrical counterpart, the way was paved for the discovery and benefits of logarithms.

It is not only in mathematics or physics that these fruitful exercises in meaning occur. Let me cite three such changes in medicine, the latter two of which have occurred in my own professional lifetime.

Example 10.9. In the nineteenth century, it was believed that a necessary (even a "normal") part of healing of a wound was suppuration. It was taken as a sign of a healthy reaction by the body; it was even called "laudable pus." A generation of surgeons was scandalized at the idea that the pus was in no way laudable and that much healthier healing and sounder scars are to be expected if suppuration can be prevented altogether.

Example 10.10. When I was a medical student, general anesthetics were directed to achieve three goals: to prevent pain; to prevent shock; and (for abdominal operations especially) to produce muscle relaxation. Specific muscle relaxants were found to achieve the last goal admirably. I can remember attending a lecture by Dr. Cecil Gray (one of the pioneers) suggesting that muscle relaxants and light anesthesia would suffice for all abdominal operations. And I can recall the reactions of many surgeons present that they were not going to risk having their patients die of shock from light anesthesia.

Example 10.11. It was the classic teaching of Welch (84) that sluggish bloodflow is one of the three cardinal causes of thrombosis. There is no doubt that thrombosis does occur preferentially in immobilized patients. But the discerning critic will raise the question of *why these patients have come to be immobilized* and what other disturbances are occurring at the same time, with which effects could be confounded. To slight this question is to agree to guilt by association. If a group of athletes were to stay in bed for six weeks, would they too be at undue risk of thrombosis? I doubt that the experiment has ever been done, or ever will be. But people resting long in bed consist largely of those in states (recovering from trauma or operations or childbirth) in which there are many radical changes, including destruction of tissue (a rich source of the clotting factor thromboplastin), that might be as plausible a culprit as low blood flow. In the early 1950s drugs that powerfully lower blood pressure were introduced. There was much concern that drugs that lower blood flow should not be used, especially in those with evidence of cerebrovascular disease. Just how wrong this opinion was has been shown since then (85, 86), despite the arguments raised to forbid such studies being done. Yet, many would ask, what mere mortal may dare call into question the edicts laid down on the basis of the opinions of Welch?

THE MEANING OF MEASURES

Against this broad background of meaning, let us turn to the problem of what we are to make of measurement. It is wise to proceed cautiously and not to be carried away by insouciant speculation.

Self-Warranted Measures

The measurement may be its own meaning, because it carries its own implications. We have seen several examples such as blood pressure in the preceding chapter in which the risk or the esthetic price is directly related to the reading itself. In cases of this kind I have argued that to intrude some spurious term (such as *hyperten-*

sion) merely confuses, and often coarsens, the understanding of the data.

Measurement and Correspondence

The meaning of measurement in commensurable entities (i.e., entities measurable in the same terms) may be that it is a gauge of correspondence between the two.

Example 10.12. The meaning of measuring for a suit of clothes may be that it provides a way of ensuring that the suit will fit. *Measurement* here is a conjunction that sets up a correspondence between the customer and the clothes. There are plenty of appliances used in medicine that it is convenient to stock in standard sizes.

In dentistry, in brace-fitting, and in making plaster casts, the fitting is done by direct molding, without the intervention of any measurement. This latter technique is expensive in time and skilled help, and is to be avoided wherever reasonable. Besides, one could reasonably send a set of measurements by telephone or radio, but scarcely a physical cast.

Measure and Adequation

The measurement may be taken as a gauge of the adequation of things that are *incommensurable,* that is, not naturally expressible on a common scale. In legal compensation by money for pain, disability, or disfigurement, one attempts to set a rate between these very different things. Such problems are often difficult to solve.

Example 10.13. We have pointed out (35) that incommensurability is a major aspect in genetic counseling where the burden—financial, emotional, and social—imposed by a disease is to be considered with the risk and weighed against the prospective benefit of having normal children. All three components (burden, risk, and benefit) are quite disparate. Even so, both the gains and the losses are shared by the parents and society, two very different kinds of measures, and by no means in fixed proportions. Even this problem is not a simple issue.

There is a deplorable lack of serious analysis of the fundamentals of this class of problems, a lack which reveals a distorted emphasis in medicine. It is only too easy to shrug one's shoulders and say that the problem is not a scientific one, or to neglect everything except the cruder costs such as hospital bills and days lost from work. Scientific or not, adequation is a real problem and one that can and shall, in fact, be solved—a responsibility often boldly assumed by those who are much less well-informed than clinicians.

Sometimes there is a reasonable empirical measure of the adequation. Whatever misgiving we might have about tests of personality, for instance, in practice they are often sound ways of identifying subjects suitable to be airline pilots, machine operators, or soldiers. They may even have professional value in recognizing which clinicians are suited to careers in research and which are not. The empirical yardstick would be how often such predictions mislead, just as an art of weather forecasting has been developed and tested.

Measurement as Evidence

The meaning of the measurement may be more subtle. It may be seen, not as something in its own right (as in the self-warranted measurement) or as a permanent medium of exchange (as in the previous section), but as a temporary structure on the way to crystallizing a concept. This use is both complicated and treacherous, and since it has an important role in medicine, it merits some careful discussion.

To focus attention, let us take a recurrent problem. We find empirically that a population of observations shows evidence of sorting itself out more or less perfectly into two groups. Two familiar examples may be cited.

Example 10.14. A histogram of single readings gathered from many people sampled from a population may exhibit two modes, i.e., there are two peaks or local maxima (fig. 10.3). Such a pattern is widely taken as manifest evidence that the population sampled is a mixture of two kinds of people, one kind clustered around each peak.

Example 10.15. In an electrophoresis there may be two distinct and well-circumscribed spots. This pattern is commonly taken to mean that there are two (probably homogeneous) compounds present with different electrical charges, so that they move at different speeds.

What are we to make of such findings? Do they mean that there are indeed two subpopulations of people and two populations of molecules respectively?

One simple answer is that there is nothing to stop us *defining* them as two populations if we want to. We may call them high and low, or fast and slow, or hyper- and hypo-. But we get nothing for nothing. Such solutions to problems by means of definitions have no merit beyond an (often empty) categorization: they guarantee no properties other than those by which we have defined them. (That does not necessarily make arbitrary definitions useless. As we

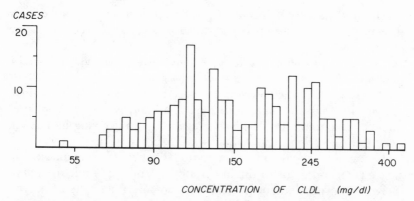

Figure 10.3. In this histogram it is arguable that there are two modes roughly in the neighborhoods of 110 and 245. Such patterns without further evidence (e.g., genetic) are often, but precariously, taken as showing that two populations are represented in the sample. The data here were given to me by Dr. P. O. Kwiterovich on the cholesterol content of low-density lipoprotein. (For purely technical reasons, the horizontal scale is logarithmic, which accounts for the uneven spacing of the values shown.)

saw in discussing self-warrant, the value itself may be the point of the point. The problems of being a dwarf, and of being a giant, are quite distinct. But clearly if what their value may be has no warrant from other sources, it will have to be judged on its future performance. Either way the arbitrary definition is apt to be a piece of temporary logical scaffolding.)

The deeper question is whether one may legitimately infer, from the two peaks and nothing more, that there are two underlying populations, homogeneous within themselves, with differences between the populations in some respect other than the characteristics we started with. The brief answer (11) is no: evidence of such grouping is neither a necessary nor a sufficient condition to establish that there is a mixture of two distributions. What then? The investigator is, in general, wise to see the presence of two peaks or spots as grounds for suspecting that there may be a mixture. This advisedly tentative surmise gains in strength if there is supporting evidence that lies quite outside the data. For instance, the transmission of the type from parent to child may follow Mendel's laws over several generations, which implies that there is some underlying factor that is holding the trait together. One such example that we have met previously is von Willebrand's disease (49). Again, detailed further chemical analysis may show that the two spots on the electrophoresis correspond to two distinct chemical compounds. In other instances the two concentrations of cases in the histogram may also prove to differ in sex, in age, in occupation, or in race.

• *The two peaks should be seen as hinting that there is a mixture; it would be perilous to see them as giving a final answer.*

There are statisticians who are prepared to try to reach a final answer by analysis alone, and there is a controversial area of numerical taxonomy (that I myself regard with misgiving because it seems to me scientifically shallow). To point to the many weaknesses in the argument from bimodality would demand much space (11), and many of the illustrations would be beside the point here. However, we may at least show how pertinent the measurements are in trying to analyze the evidence that there is a mixture.

Measurement enters at two points: in the construction of the measure itself and in the genesis of the distribution. For no special reason (other than familiarity) we shall illustrate some of these ideas with the Gaussian (normal) distribution.

The Genesis of the Measurement. Surprisingly often, a measurement devised outside the CGS scale turns out to have been devised because of the demands imposed by data.

Example 10.16. The classical example is the so-called intelligence quotient, which is a scale of performance constructed out of arbitrarily chosen data in such a way as to give a Gaussian distribution. This solution involved an artificial weighting of the representation and scores for the various components of intelligence examined in the test. The test has been used for so long that one is apt to forget the highly nonformal nature of its origin; but occasionally the results from applying such tests seem to be so anomalous as to raise questions in critical minds. (Differences in intelligence scores among racial groups and the controversy that ensued are a striking example.)

Example 10.17. Let us go through an imaginary exercise to illustrate the difficulties in devising and interpreting a new scheme of measurement. The very way in which we try to think of any trait tends to yield a kind of bell-shaped distribution. We commonly think of most people as being mediocre (M) or ordinary or regular. On the one side, a smaller number are gifted or talented (T), many of them earmarked for advanced education; and on the other side, another minor group are deprived (D) or handicapped, and many of them have to be maintained in institutions. A much smaller group are those extraordinary people who find their way into newspapers—the geniuses (G), the fastest this, the tallest that; while at the other extreme are those so incapacitated (I) as to require extraordinary care and who furnish the "human interest" stories in newspapers. Now the numbers that fall into the various classes are also constrained. There can never be a great number of exceptional cases* or (rather obviously) they would not be exceptional. So the two extreme groups are necessarily small. The numbers that can be taken care of in institutions or that can profit from advanced studies are ruthlessly kept small by economics. We could not live in a society in which most people are not mediocre. So we have a pattern much like that shown in figure 10.4A. The main force determining this pattern is, as it were, the solidarity of the mediocre. However, there are two common counterforces to it.

The first is that the mediocre compete among themselves and tend to make much of what differences there are among them, differences that to the very intelligent or the very dull may be barely perceptible. The mediocre people do all the ordinary jobs, and since there are preferences (real or imagined) among such jobs, those competing may devise many shades of differences in their endowments and credentials, in a fashion that the extraordinary people do not; and since it is often the mediocre who decide on standards, the measurement in the middle tends to be stretched out in the interests of discernment, and the same number of people are spaced over a wider, artificially expanded section. (This will not happen if the measurement has a firm objective basis, as height and body weight do. But we are concerned with the case where the measurement is being invented.) It is rather like stretching a piece of toffee between the fingers until it thins at some point in the middle. The area (probability) in the distribution, like the volume of toffee, must be kept constant throughout. The concentration is lessened in the center and there may even develop two peaks, one in each understretched part (fig. 10.4B). This change could never happen if the measurement were something in itself apart from the data, e.g., a measurement of distance or weight. By contrast, if none of these forces was at work, the measure would be a matter of percentiles and have the bland form of fig. 10.4C.

A second mechanism reinforces this spurious grouping: polarization. Thus, while political opinion may in fact show a continuous range, individuals tend to identify themselves as, say, the conservatives and suppose that they have nothing in common with the radicals. For instance, at one time, the psychologists distinguished *introverts* from *extroverts;* and later, type A personalities were

*Compare Lord Melbourne's comment to Queen Victoria: "There are not many very good anything" (87).

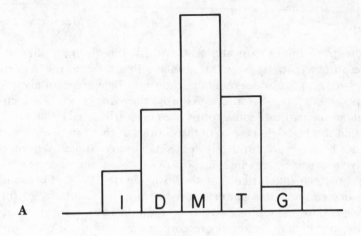

A

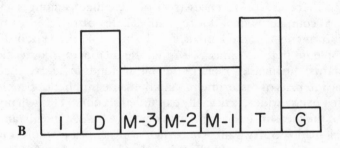

B

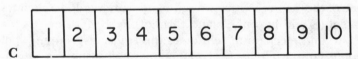

C

Figure 10.4. Bimodality produced in a graded variable with no established scale of measurement. *A:* The habitual pattern of thought (that most people are ordinary and the atypical cases less common) tends to produce a unimodal distribution. *B:* However, rivalry and polarization in the mediocre (which leads to uneven stretching of the scale of assessment) may lead to thinning of the central section so that by comparison the others tend to become modes. This phenomenon would not occur if the metric were defined independently of the grouping. *C:* This distribution would result when the values are grouped by the deciles (each of them one-tenth of the distribution).

thought to be at high risk of coronary disease, whereas the type B's were not. Further experience suggested that both polarizations were artificial. Geneticists at first accepted the common notion that there are blue-eyed and brown-eyed people and red-headed people, traits that were even thought at one stage to be Mendelian; subsequent analysis of quantitative measurements on them (88, 89) showed that the borderline cases so far outnumber the true types that it became impossible to believe that they are authentic categories.

The reader might suppose that these odd results are produced only by subjectivism and prejudice, but such is not the case. In the first place, it is arguable that in the last paragraph I have overstepped my warrant. I say, for instance, that belief in "red hair" as a distinct natural category was discredited by objective measurements. But by what right do I overtrump the esthetic opinions of (say) Titian by quantitative measurements? Would we accept the notion that the opinions of Ruskin can be demolished by measuring the sizes of the paintings that he analyzed? This is a serious objection, which it is by no means easy to answer. For there are without doubt rare skills (in wine tasting, for instance) that have been convincingly tested by empirical studies. They are not to be discredited either by the indifference of vulgar taste or by coarse (if "objective") chemical gauges. I could be convinced that there is a particular color of Titian red hair if it could be unvaryingly identified by a fixed competent class of observers on extensive testing.

Consider a more vexed problem of the quantitation. At first it may appear trivial. If we were to grade paintings by size, should we use length or area?

Example 10.18. To be less exotic, suppose we wish to see whether in some patients there are two classes of red blood cells, to be distinguished by their sizes. Should we look at diameters? Or areas? Or volumes? One may suppose that it does not make much difference. But it does. It has been known for many years that if a measurement has a single mode, the measurement raised to a power, even a fraction of a power, may be bimodal (90). And for those who (in the teeth of my warning) regard bimodality as the infallible bench mark of heterogeneity, what conclusion they arrive at may depend even on which choice they make to represent the measurement.

Example 10.19. Suppose that a column source of light has a central area of high illumination (a focus) and the illumination it gives has some scatter at the edges. When it is projected on a circular screen, the intensity of the light follows (say) a Gaussian distribution (fig. 10.5, bottom). But that part of the light projected above

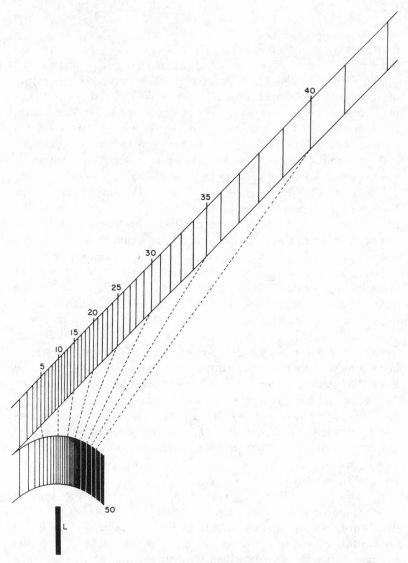

Figure 10.5. The intensity of the light from a column source of light (*L*). Part of the light is thrown on a semicircular screen and has a Gaussian distribution. The vertical lines there represent the 1, 2, . . . 50 percentiles. Their closeness is an indication of the probability density. Because they become so crowded in the center, every fifth percentile is shown in white. The top part of the light shines over the top of the screen down a long street. Corresponding percentiles are connected by dashed lines. The central part of the distribution is stretched because of the increasing obliquity of the light to the walls of the houses in the street. The uneven stretching means that at first there is a crowding of percentiles and then a progressive spacing out. The half of the distribution on the left side of the street is shown here. The other half will have a corresponding spread on the right. The distribution of intensity plotted against distance will have two modes, one for the negative angles (on the left) and one for positive angles (on the right).

the screen shines down an infinitely long straight street (fig. 10.5, top). The light it sheds on the face of any one house depends on two factors. The houses illuminated by the more central part of the beam tend to have the strongest source of light, but since they are also the most distant, the effect of the light is diluted because it is striking their faces more and more obliquely. So with gradually increasing distance, the illumination first builds up (because the light is coming from progressively nearer the focus) and then falls (because of the increasing obliquity). The same pattern will be followed on the other side of the street. Thus, the distribution becomes clearly bimodal. By extension of this argument, it is easily enough shown that under certain plausible conditions (and for this very reason) *the ratio of two Gaussian variates may have two modes* and may be erroneously taken to mean that there is heterogeneity, whereas it is the resultant of these two conflicting trends (centrality and obliquity).

• *To use the ratio of two random numbers as an index is a task best left to the mathematical statistician.*

Yet I could make a long and painful list of ratios that are used in every branch of medicine (including dosages) in which this peril is blithely ignored. It is no wonder that reputations are so often made by demolishing other people's indiscretions.

A REHABILITATION

In spite of all these problems, we must not turn our backs on measurement. The twin coinages of science are counting and measurement. Their relative standings vary from time to time. In genetics, for instance, between 1918 and 1945 measurement had a major, perhaps an unhealthily dominating role; since 1945 the reaction to this domination has undermined the hegemony to the point that the main concern of genetics is currently thought to be the classification of pure compounds. I have no doubt that there will be a counterreaction in time. A common view holds to the primacy of classes and treats measurement as a mere attribute (91). Which (if either) is the ultimate basis of scientific understanding, I cannot say; but I think it would be wise to treat them as though on an equal footing. There are cases where each of them will break down.

That thought is cold comfort to those wondering what they should respect and believe. I would recommend that one should never abdicate one's reason to measurement, most especially when there are any grounds for doubting the credentials or the impartiality (conscious or unconscious) of the person who devised the measurement. Measurement is one of the major currencies of science, but more often than not it is to be seen as a means and not an end. It stands or falls by how it improves understanding and by the discoveries to which it leads. It is evidence, but only part of the evidence. How is it to be gauged? Let me suggest several criteria.

Measurement as a Means to Isolating Entities

The measurement may lead to finding classes that eventually prove to have distinguishing features other than the measurement itself. The classes may, as we have seen, represent chemical differences (like the electrophoretic mobility of various hemoglobins), or traits that have been conserved over many generations, as in von Willebrand's disease (49).

One should not dismiss the measurement as of no further interest once an underlying class has been unearthed by it. Measurements in women of some feature of an X-linked trait such as hemophilia may help more or less to decide *whether she is a carrier.* The class to which she belongs is the principal issue for genetic counseling; but *for her own prognosis* it is the measurement itself that matters, and some carriers may have higher levels of factor VIII than some noncarriers. What is transmitted is genotype; what matters, for the personal fitness, is phenotype. That simple contrast, in the present emphasis on reductionist genetics, is apt to be overlooked altogether.

Measurement and Prognosis

The measurement may or may not show its worth by what its prognostic implications are. Body temperature, for instance, has importance in its own right: the body could not long withstand a temperature of 110°F. It has prognostic significance; but it is by no means a simple relationship. A temperature of 103°F would not be very unusual in lobar pneumonia; it would be frightening in appendicitis. Sometimes it is not the level but the variation in the temperature that is the main significant point (e.g., in tertian malaria).

Measurement and Relationship

Measurement may be important as a method of showing a correspondence between features, and hence it may either improve our understanding of mechanisms (for instance, between intracellular potassium concentration and the level of bicarbonate in the plasma) or eliminate the need for redundant, or almost redundant, measurements.

Example 10.20. The degree of maturity of the skeleton, "the bone age," as judged by X-ray of the wrist, is highly correlated with assessment by X-rays of other bones; and from the point of view of risk to the patient, it is much to be preferred to an X-ray of the pelvis.

Heuristic Value of Measurement

In the long run, at least, the interest of a measurement depends on the discoveries and the insight that it contributes. This criterion is difficult to assess; but as in Darwinian selection, time determines the sense of usefulness.

Example 10.21. Vital capacity (the volume of the maximum breath one can take and exhale), though an admirably precise and reproducible test, is now thought to be of little interest in investigating respiratory disease, largely because it takes no account of the rate at which respiratory gases can be exchanged.

Example 10.22. Measuring the basal metabolic rate is now gone quite out of fashion, because it is cumbersome and difficult to standardize, and is at best an indirect test of thyroid function.

This process of editing tests is a slow one; and when we deplore the number of futile measurements there are in current use in Medicine, perhaps we should realize how much more complicated biology is than physics, how much less well-defined the topics are, and how short the tradition of quantitative medicine.

RESOLVING POWER, PRECISION, AND ACCURACY

So far, we have dealt with judging of measurement from the outside: how it matches up with our understanding beyond the measurement itself. It is worthwhile to say something about the internal properties, if for no other reason than that their importance is incorrectly stressed. There are three properties that are commonly confused that we shall address (11).

Resolving Power

The nature of a system will often dictate the limits of nicety of a measurement.

Example 10.23. It is well known that by light microscopy one cannot distinguish two points that are less than about 0.2μ apart: one cannot see a structure of any smaller size. This limit is inexorably set by the shortest wavelength of visible light.

Sometimes resolving power is determined by the fineness of calibration available, a feature determined by the manufacturer. Most observers can, and will, interpolate between markings, but it takes an unusual eye to do so reliably to less than one-tenth of a unit.

From a clinical standpoint, the limit of resolution may be set by the indefiniteness of the issue. Suppose a cardiologist wishes to time how quickly pain develops on effort in a patient with angina pectoris. The dividing points between a strange sensation and discomfort or between discomfort and frank pain may be such as to make any exact statement impossible; the resolving power will not be improved if an ordinary watch is replaced by an atomic clock calibrated in thousandths of a second.

Example 10.24. Lewis (92) furnished an excellent clinical example. The limits of a lobar pneumonia can be mapped out more or less accurately by percussion, a means of examination that yields a difference in resonance between healthy and affected tissue. Ordinarily, the heart gives a duller sound than the lung; and in the past this method was used to determine the size of the heart. However, Lewis pointed out that the heart—having a globular shape in all directions, but no edges—recedes gradually from the chest wall with a widening wedge of lung intervening. This relationship means that there is a gradually increasing resonance (fig. 10.6A). Attempts to define the limits of the heart by percussion are looking for a sharp transition in resonance that does not exist. If, as sometimes happens, the heart is so large as to push the lung aside and leave a wide area of direct contact with the chest wall (and hence of dulness), one may be able to recognize that the heart is enlarged even if there is still no way of sharply defining its limits (fig. 10.6B). But in most hearts, percussion is of little value.

We may note two important features of resolving power.

First, it need not, and often will not, involve any authentic random component whatsoever.

Example 10.25. How closely I may measure a pupil, with a scale calibrated in centimeters, has nothing to do with random variation in the intensity of the light which influences the size of the pupil. Of course, the observer may read the scale erroneously. But even the infallible observer can make no more exact statement than that the measurement certainly lies between two calibration marks on the scale. It is the size of this interval of markings that tells us what the resolving power of the method is and how the results should be expressed.

Second, other things being equal, the higher the resolving power, the better. But a measurement with a high resolving power may, in the particular case, be of little use.

Example 10.26. Height (measured to however many significant

A

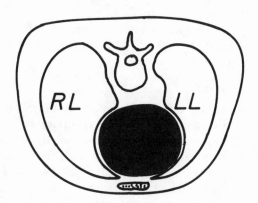

B

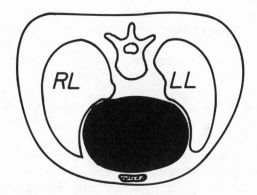

Figure 10.6. The indefiniteness of delimitation of the heart by percussion. *A:* View, from above, of a transverse section of the thorax, showing why it is hard to delimit the heart by percussion. Note the globular shape of the heart (*in black*) and its complete lack of edges; the gradual intrusion of an increasing thickness of lung between the heart and the chest wall as we go laterally; and how far the chest wall is from the extreme lateral borders of the heart. *B:* Here the heart is enlarged, and the area in contact with the chest wall (which gives a dull note on percussion) will be increased; but the limits will still be indefinite and imperfectly related to the width of the heart. (The dotted mass in front of (here, below) the heart is the sternum [breast bone]. RL = right lung; LL = left lung.)

figures) tells us little about intelligence. Conversely, one can tell a dwarf from a giant with the unaided eye.

The criterion of resolving power is the interval of uncertainty, and it is commonly written thus: 27 ± 0.5 mm, meaning the limits 26.5 mm and 27.5 mm.

Precision

This term is usefully applied only to those measurements in which random variation is of at least comparable size to the limit of uncertainty. The error of measurement or the spontaneous variation in the value must be large enough that there is at least a moderate risk of the observed value lying in either (or any) of at least two intervals in the calibrated scale.

Precision, then, means how reproducible results are. Usually it is an easy quality to evaluate: for instance, by multiple determinations of what purports to be the same quantity. If there are big discrepancies among the results, even on two aliquots from the same sample, the method is imprecise. The significance of high precision is overrated. A method may be precise, but precisely wrong. The baseline setting may be faulty; or a standard reference solution may be inappropriate; yet the measurements may remain highly reproducible.

The criterion of precision of a result is its standard deviation.*
• *One does not indicate the precision by the number of significant figures in the result.*

To say that a sample mean is 21.4 does *not* mean that the true mean is certain to lie between 21.35 and 21.45. One can infer nothing about precision from the point estimate 21.4. The appropriate expression would be of the form "21.4; s.d. = 2.1." Many brought up to think in terms of resolving power suppose that if the imprecision is so great, then the sample mean should be expressed as 21, or even "about 20." But it is easily shown that *this kind of rounding makes the statement even more incorrect.* There is no necessary relationship between precision and resolving power at all. But in dealing with *any quantity that involves any mathematical manipulation at all beyond straightforward measurement,* it is best to treat the result as if random and not to express its refinement by the number of decimal places. (Of course, an unreasonable number of decimal places may offend against one's sense of scientific style. But that is a matter of taste, not of ironclad principle.)

---

*The estimated standard deviation of the estimate is commonly and confusingly referred to as the standard error. I try to avoid this latter term altogether, which seems to cause nothing but trouble.

Accuracy

A measure is accurate *if its performance on average* is close to the true value to be determined. That is no guarantee that it is precise, or conversely.

Example 10.27. Suppose, for instance, that we wish to determine the mean height of all males in Baltimore. To do so, I propose to take a strict probability sample of two men, measure their heights competently with an inch tape, and average them. We are quite sure that the prescription for getting the result is an accurate estimator of the true mean, but an imprecise one. If, using an interferometer, I measure the heights in five thousand boys attending pediatric hospitals, the average will be highly precise, but (since by no stretch of imagination are boys in a pediatric hospital representative of all boys) it will be inaccurate, perhaps highly so.

In general, it is much harder to assess accuracy than precision. Indeed, there are many instances where we cannot determine it, since for one reason or another the true value cannot be found. For instance, a quantity may be measurable only by a technique involving an intervention that may seriously change the quantity of interest.

Example 10.28. As we noted previously, the oldest way to measure cerebral blood flow is by having the subject inhale a foreign gas while blood is sampled through needles inserted into the jugular bulb (68). These procedures may very well change cerebral blood flow (because of nervousness or overbreathing). Then we may more or less readily measure the precision of the method, but we have no way of knowing what the results would be like if we were not doing the procedure. In such cases, one must be content to make comparisons (among people or between readings in the same subject) supposing the same set of biases to be operating in all cases. More modern methods involve external imaging after inhaling radioactive xenon. They are less disturbing, and I have some assurance that they are more accurate.

The criterion of accuracy is bias: how much discrepancy there will be on average between the mean value of the estimate and the true value it is designed to estimate. Sometimes the bias is expressed as a quantity, sometimes as a percentage of the true value.

PROBLEMS

10.1. Consider the resolving power, the precision, and the accuracy of the following measurements:

    a. The intelligence quotient in a student in nursery school (prekindergarten)

b. The age of a person picked at random
c. The size of the stomach in a living patient
d. The effect on the brain of a drug given by mouth.

10.2. Analyze the meaning of the following measurements:
a. The size of the brain
b. The average volume of the lungs
c. The peripheral resistance (= the mean blood pressure divided by the cardiac output).

10.3. Consider the heuristic value of the following ideas:
a. Homeostasis
b. Darwinian fitness
c. Stress
d. Suffering
e. Identity.

10.4. Consider the following argument: "A statement cannot be said to be true if it cannot even in principle be proved to be false if it is false. But from symmetry, a statement cannot be said to be false if it cannot even in principle be proved to be true if it is true. Then perhaps some statements cannot be said to be either true or false." Apply this argument to the topic of free will.

10.5. Data are presented in a graph showing the relationship between the cardiac output in liters per minute per square meter body surface against a dose of digoxin in milligrams per kilogram body weight. (The surface area is computed from an empirical formula based on the product of the height and weight raised to fractional powers.) Identify what exactly is being displayed in this diagram.

10.6. The radius of a circle is known by comparison against an exact scale to be between 9 and 10 mm. What limits can one set on the area of the circle? Justify the terms of your answer. ($\pi = 3.1415926535\ldots$)

10.7. The mean of twenty-five measurements on the radius of a circle is 9.492 mm, and the standard deviation of the result is known from theory to be 0.038. Assuming the results are normally distributed, find as accurately as possible 95 percent confidence limits on the true value.

10.8. If a patient *feels* happy, does that mean that the patient *is* happy?

11 | Modeling

Here and there in the earlier parts of this book, we have touched on the notions and uses of modeling. In this chapter I shall try to confront the issues directly and to set them in perspective. All science ultimately embodies two complementary and, at times, conflicting demands: empirical fact and orderly conjecture. While it endures, their union provides excitement, enrichment, fecundity. There is a perpetual risk of disruption with harmful consequences to the well-being of the products. If the history of science tells us anything worthwhile, it is that, even if the occasional foray into pure theory or pure data collection adds spice to enquiry, final estrangement can only corrupt.

As to the one extreme, as Whitehead (26) points out, the corruption of medieval science lay in the neglect of empirical fact.

Example 11.1. As late as the seventeenth century Galileo's fellow scholars were trying to overtrump his observations on the shape of the moon's surface with arguments based on what theory says its shape should be. Much fun has been poked at their attempts to ascribe the bumps and hollows he saw on it to flaws in his system of lenses. But an argument (however weak) that is intended seriously demands a serious answer: one does not learn to become a scholar by making fun of other scholars. For the unmellowed antithesis of one heresy is always another heresy. While by their whole stance Galileo's critics showed an undue emphasis on theory, they nevertheless can be applauded for two features for which they have not received fair treatment by the pamphleteers.

First, they are right in that celestial bodies do have shapes that can be formulated by theory and could be explained, for instance, by the mechanics of a rotating molten body (about which of course, they knew little). If an astronomer were to observe a large cubical body in space, he would have every reason to believe, on the grounds of shape alone, that it was not an authentic planet. Galileo's dispute with his colleagues was not about large-scale shape but about *surface* characteristics. These characteristics are what they are (as like as not, because of random accidents); and they are to be discovered by looking. But it would not be totally incongruous for the scientist to invoke theory when considering the shape of a celestial body.

Second, while I cannot vouch for their motives, Galileo's critics were right to call into question the properties of a new method of observation, especially when it was leading to radically new conclusions for which, at the time, there were no independent means of corroboration. Doubtless a later critic would propose to explore the point by examining how the telescope behaves when used on distant terrestrial objects that could be subsequently examined. But the discrepancies that would certainly come to light would be patched up by appealing to atmospheric pollution, thermal irregularities (shimmer), and temperature gradients (mirages, etc.). On these terms, it is only in the last few years that there has been any way of testing by direct corroborative observation what the properties of light propagated over a quarter of a million miles are. The supercilious dabblers if challenged would find it much harder to justify our present confidence in the data of light astronomy than they might suppose.*

Popper (93) shows the absurdity of the other extreme, the notion, espoused by Francis Bacon, that the scientist may usefully observe the empirical world without context or without any sense that what one observes has any immediate need to be fitted together. There results a thesis that there is, as it were, a conceptual glue that holds our ideas together, a glue that is something other than the things themselves. This sense of coherence as separate from the facts themselves pervades Medicine. Whatever fire it comes under from the theorists, for us clinicians it seems to be indispensible to coherent thought.

Example 11.2. The diagnostic process characteristically consists of hearing symptoms and soliciting *pertinent* details about them; examining the patient with *selective* emphasis; and carrying out *appropriate* further investigations. Some clinicians of Baconian tem-

---

*I do not put myself on the side of Galileo's critics and their excessive and destructive criticism. Nevertheless, I would not abdicate my right to dissect a new idea simply because they may have abused theirs.

per teach their students that they should "let the patient tell his own story in his own words" and then "examine the patient from head to toe." They say that "if after doing so, the physician does not know the diagnosis, the history and examination should be repeated and extended." Now there is a metaphorical truth in these maxims, which are sentiments designed to encourage perceptiveness and thoroughness. But none of them can possibly be taken literally. To examine the entire patient thoroughly, scrutinize the nervous system in minute detail, search every centimeter of skin with a hand lens, test every muscle and joint, elicit every physical sign that has ever been described, would take hours, perhaps days; and the attentive cooperation of a patient (especially of a sick one) soon falters. A full history, which would include everything in the patient's past life, would take months and result in a full-scale biography. (A detailed psychoanalysis would take years of hard work.) As to bedside diagnosis, if this were to be secure without special tests, in many cases it would come far too late for effective treatment. Yet again, to do every conceivable test, leaving expense and danger aside, would take so long that treatment that depended on the diagnosis being made first would have to be postponed indefinitely.

All these activities must be seen in perspective, and we should heed the words in italics: *pertinent, selective, appropriate.* The difficulty is to prescribe how these processes are to operate. If the diagnosis were known at the start, one would know what data are to the point. But this last statement is a tacit recognition that the diagnosis is something other than the evidence on which it is made. If it were not so, then, pushing it to the extreme, the diagnostic process would amount to nothing more than finding out what data on the patient were remarkable. In particular, the traditional concerns of the clinician—"What disease does the patient have?" and "How many diseases does the patient have?"—would no longer have any evident meaning.

The truth, I suspect, is somewhere between total amorphism and fanatical regimentation. No doubt many ominous findings mean nothing more than the findings themselves. Obesity may be a disturbing finding only in that obesity is bad for health. We have dealt at length with this matter in chapter 8. But certainly not all diagnoses have this immediacy. If it were possible to review an exhaustive set of data at leisure, sooner or later one might be able to resolve the issues of diagnosis in the patient. But the diagnostician does not have an indefinite amount of time; and in deciding what selected information to seek, the answer obviously cannot be based on knowing all the facts, because the issue is precisely which of these facts we should try to acquire. This almost paradoxical quality makes it difficult to formulate the nature of the diagnostic process. It is akin to what, in the context of scientific enquiry, I earlier called illation.

It would be a mistake, however, to see the diagnostic process as unique in this respect. For this very same paradox underlies all medical research, and indeed, I suspect, all scholarship. If the scholar knew the answer, he would know what evidence he needed to find the answer; but if he knew the answer, he would not need to obtain the evidence. How is this puzzle to be solved? In the writings of many, there is a strong, almost mystical, sense about how discoveries are made. Popper, citing an address by Einstein (94 p. 32), seems to say little more than that one cannot write prescriptions for genius; Kuhn (70) distinguishes between ordinary solving of mundane problems inside an orthodox framework of "paradigms" (an activity that he calls "normal science") and rare transcendent insights, such as Newton's gravitation, in which the paradigms themselves are modified ("scientific revolutions"). Both writers have a valuable insight; but both (in my opinion from inside Medicine) make rather too much of it. It seems to me that Kuhn (a physicist and a historian of science) characterizes these revolutions both by their originality and boldness on the one hand and by the far-reaching consequences that they have in science on the other. It is not hard to think of hundreds of minor, but ingenious, discoveries (in Medicine or Nursing, for instance) that have a narrow area of application. Many represent intuitive leaps that can by no stretching of words be represented as a gradual evolution or a deduction from what went before.

Example 11.3. There is nothing in the least like a medical precursor for the use of curare as a muscle relaxant in abdominal surgery.* There have since been extensive elaborations of it. I am sure that it has saved more lives than cardiac transplants have.

Example 11.4. The same might be said of putting iodine in table salt to prevent endemic goiter, once a disfiguring disease, which is now virtually extinct.

I daresay Kuhn would not rate either as scientific revolutions. Yet despite the modest leaps involved in both cases, neither can be seen as "normal science" in the sense that they represent mechan-

---

*Previous attempts to increase muscle relaxation were based on deeper anesthesia (which was dangerous and involved no selective local action at all) and intercostal block (which was not systemic and called for unusual technical skill).

ical applications of established methods or even that the idea embodied in each (as distinct from the means for implementing it) could be deduced from a secure set of axioms.

One can make altogether too much out of the melodramatic quality of discovery; and it is only too easy for the journalist, concerned with writing "a good story" about the discovery, to tell the tale with artificial highlights and unsound emphases. It is from such journalistic portrayals that those absurd and distasteful controversies arise about whether the calculus was invented by Newton or Leibniz, impressionism by Turner or Monet, the prevention of sepsis by Semmelweiss or Lister or Holmes.

As to the stance that one cannot write blueprints for genius, it does not seem to me a helpful statement in any way. It is a truism without being a truth. Of course, to have devised a profound formula converts a cluster of major discoveries into a set of applications.

Example 11.5. Once Selyi introduced the idea of stress as a cause of disease (95), countless lesser minds seized on it and made a fashion of it.

But to view all intuitive jumps as Kuhnian misleads by its undue emphasis on changes of heroic proportions. It is rare (if it ever happens at all) that a major and disruptive discovery comes as a blinding flash of insight; rather it is the cumulative effect of a great many sparks. Sanger's work on the structure of insulin took ten years; Newton's theory of gravitation took twenty; the therapeutic application of penicillin by Cheyne and Florey from Fleming's original note took fourteen. These revolutions were mainly the result of sustained hard work, intellectual courage, and repeated exercise of minor ingenuities. While these hard facts are matters much more for the career scientist than for my readers (and certainly merit the attentions of the historian), nevertheless they should help to keep a sense of balance. A new idea is neither good because it is new nor bad because it is not yet a fact. Novelty is merely such a small part of a discovery that it must be judged by what it leads to, and not by its attractiveness alone. Knowing which idea to follow, and how far, is the difficult part of discovery; but that art can, and must, be cultivated.

THE NOTION OF A MODEL

Discovery in Medicine, then, is a balance between surmise and empirical fact, neither of which can thrive indefinitely in isolation. Elsewhere (96) I have compared the relationship between them to that between the tent poles and the tent. Without the canvas (which is like being without the facts), one has no equipment for confronting harsh reality. The tent poles alone do not protect one against the rain, nor does endless thinking meet all our concrete needs. But equally, an unshaped huddle of canvas, like a haphazard assembly of facts, fails in its main purpose of giving shelter. Neither structure can meet both needs. Surmise guides, empirical fact gives warrant.

A major problem in discussing models is the ambiguity of the term. It is used in many senses to mean many things, often only feebly related to each other. For our present purposes, we may distinguish among three types.

The Biologist's Model

The biologist approaches surmise with an allegiance to actual or supposed concrete realities. Thus, he must begin with a "cast of characters" fashioned out of accumulated experiences in the field, cautiously and sparingly discarded, or added to, from time to time. The list will naturally depend on the field involved.

Example 11.6. A pathologist may start out with a belief in inflammation, the various types of leucocytes, phagocytosis, antibodies, chemotaxis, and so forth. They are stable, but not immutable, structures of thought. For instance, there has been much written on just how many distinct types of white cells there are, what the chemicals are that provoke inflammation, and so forth. The pathologist's sense of the reality of these structures comes from observation, by naked eye and by microscope, aided more or less artificially by the use of dyes, fluorescent antibodies, and the like.

Example 11.7. The expert on infectious disease and epidemics thinks in terms of infecting organisms; channels through which they are spread (direct contact, fomites, aerial droplets); infectivity; immune, susceptible, incubating, and infectious, subjects and their movements in the population; morbidity, disablement and mortality; and so forth.

Example 11.8. The geneticist thinks of chromosomes, meiosis, mitosis, (all visible); segregation, recombination, transmission, dominance and recessivity, transcription, translation (all processes); the gene (a conceptualization); and the rest.

All these models of the biologist have a number of characteristics in common.

The Role of Imagery. They all carry mental images of what is happening, the component parts having known, or surmised, properties of their own (e.g., the physical mobilities of the various leucocytes) and properties in relationship to the others (such as the death lock between an antigen and an antibody). Some of these entities (such as chemotaxis, infectivity, dominance) may prove, on further analysis, to be redundant concepts; or after close inspection, they may prove too formless to be useful. But correct or not, the terms of discussion lie in frankly empirical matters of observation and of immediate inference from them.

Example 11.9. Mendelian segregation of traits was first an empirical fact. The existence of the gene, as it were the genetic atom, was a surmise that came half a century later; and despite intermittent euphoria in cycles of about ten years or so in which it is supposed that finally the full nature of the gene is understood, the gene remains somewhat of an enigma.

The Corroborative Role of Empiricism. The intellectual discipline applied to (as it were) regulating and licensing these biological models is empirical. The scientist spends much time in exploring how the components behave when manipulated in a particular way under certain circumstances. While responses will commonly be measured or counted, neither gauge is an integral part of the study in the sense of being indispensible. Much of cell biology and pathology owes nothing to the study of numbers or quantity.

Deductive or Inferential Character. Such models have a strictly inferential character, by which we mean that the process of reasoning goes mainly from the results of the model to principle, and not conversely. The microbiologist will of course wonder why some organisms can live in dust and others require moisture at all times; but the question is prompted after, and by, the fact that they do have these properties; and in the end, the model, however elaborated, must square with these facts if it is to be effective.

The Analogue. There is another sense in which the biologist (especially in pathology) uses the word *model*. It does not denote any kind of abstraction or conceptualization at all, but a state occurring naturally or produced, usually in an animal, that bears sufficient resemblance to a disease to be used as a means of studying and manipulating the disease. There exist neurological disorders, cancers, blood anomalies, and so on in mice that appear to be rather like familiar diseases in man; and one may, for example, try out certain drugs on them as a preliminary to using them in man. For my part, I see the term *model* in such a context something of a misnomer; I would prefer to call it an "animal analogue."

The Statistician's Model

The prime allegiance of the mathematical statistician is quite different. It lies in the behavior of systems, founded on certain axioms that can be stated before the outcomes can be known. *If* a random variable has such and such properties and a sample is collected in a certain way, *then* a particular test of hypothesis or estimator will have corresponding properties.

Example 11.10. Consider a system in which a number of events, all of one form, may occur randomly and at a constant probability from instant to instant. Moreover, suppose that what happens in the next interval, whether long or short, is in no way influenced by what has already happened, however recently or remotely in the past. Then the outcome will follow what is called the Poisson distribution. It has well-defined properties. I will not trouble the reader with details, which are purely technical and quite beside the point here (96 pp. 103 ff).

Much of the statistician's life revolves around exploring facets of the Poisson model and similar logical systems. Now it will be noted that this model has a totally different standing from the biological one. The Poisson model starts with a series of axioms (stated, rather informally, in example 11.10) from which everything else is deduced, including how to use it statistically. There is no statement as to what the events involved are that have the properties enjoyed in the statistician's model, and no associated imagery at all (both of which would, to the theorist, be merely distractions). There is not the least point in trying to see whether the deductions are true by any means other than scrutinizing the mathematics. If a set of empirical data were found to be at odds with the predictions, all one could infer is that the experiment from which the data were derived must in some way violate the set of axioms underlying the model. This conclusion is not an indictment of either the model or the experiment.

Thus, we have two models developed from different starting points and with different properties and scope, leading to different predictions.

• *There is no* necessary *relationship between these two kinds of models.*

Nevertheless, they may prove mutually enriching, often to a profound degree. But the added step of bringing them together suffers at the hands of two extremists. The one says that the two bear no relationship at all to each other. The other supposes that the adaptation of the one to the other is a trivial problem to be settled by the biologist and the statistician over a small cup of warm coffee.

The Biomathematician's Model

The matchmaker may be the biomathematician who, if he is faithful to his hybrid ancestry, is concerned with setting up correspondences between the abstract terms of the mathematics and the concrete terms of the biology. He may not merely contribute to harmony between the two but may also shed light on them separately. He may point out inconsistencies and redundancies in the way the biologist has formulated his problem. He may detect ambiguities in the way the statistician has solved it.

Biologists, for example, have a tendency to confuse *random* with *indiscriminate*. Thus, where time-dependent processes are concerned, a random end point tends to be mistaken for a system that has no memory.

Example 11.11. Most people deteriorate and die perhaps as a result of accumulated physical or chemical insults; and the death rate at age ninety is higher than it is at age ten. These facts are commonly misinterpreted in two ways. First, it is supposed that death *cannot* be a random process, since the risk of it depends on age. Second, a process called ageing is invoked to explain the changes with age; there are even vigorous schools of biology that believe that ageing is a genetically programmed phenomenon with selective advantage in the Darwinian sense. Now one cannot, without more insight, dismiss both these conclusions as false. However, a very little mathematics is enough to show that neither is a necessary belief. A search for a specific, inborn, cause of ageing *may* be a total waste of effort. It is not true that randomness demands that the mortality rate be the same at all ages. To the contrary, on a continuous time scale there is only one process (the exponential) for which that property holds. The incorrect conclusion reflects a fundamental confusion between *random* mortality and *indiscriminate* mortality. The latter is illustrated by the mortality rate in an airplane crash or a bomb explosion, which will be virtually independent of age. The key to this kind of insight is to rescue the enquiring mind from empty words used to describe ill-understood processes, words that in easy stages become endowed with a spurious entity. One throws no light whatsoever on ageing by saying that it is due to senescence.

Biology left to itself furnishes feeble guidance in marshaling a set of measurements on a patient. There is a maximum amount of information that can be extracted from them. Yet there is a common practice of juggling them in a variety of ways (which have no theoretical justification) in the hope that some penetrating truth will emerge.

Example 11.12. One simple instance is the monitoring of coagulation by the prothrombin assay. The result may be given as "prothrombin time" (the time until a fibrin clot forms when a standard source of thromboplastin is added to a particular preparation of blood). But this time is often divided into a constant (which we may denote by k) to give a "percentage of normal prothrombin level." Now insofar as the test is used to see whether an effective dosage of anticoagulant is being given, the last step is superfluous. For the objective of keeping the prothrombin time between a and b *corresponds exactly* to the objective of keeping the "prothrombin percentage" between k/a and k/b. This correspondence is like the equivalence between saying "Baltimore is one-sixth of the way from Washington to New York" and saying "Baltimore is five-sixths of the way from New York to Washington." The only effect of the second step is to furnish an opportunity to make a mistake in calculation.*

Example 11.13. Another, somewhat more elaborate and more devastating example also comes from hematology; see for example, Wintrobe et al. (97). Three measures are commonly used in assessing anemia. We shall denote them by R (the number of red cells per cubic millimeter), P (the packed-cell volume or hematocrit, i.e., the proportion by volume of the blood that is occupied by cells), and H (the concentration of hemoglobin in grams per deciliter of blood). They are often converted into three "red cell indices" (with suitable dimensions), namely, the mean corpuscular volume $(MCV) = P/R;$ the mean corpuscular hemoglobin $(MCH) = H/R;$ and the mean corpuscular hemoglobin concentration $(MCHC) = H/P$. With a little algebra, it is evident that $MCV = MCH/MCHC$, an equation that may be rearranged to express any index as a function of the other two.

What has resulted from this maneuver? First, three values have been replaced by three indices, so there is *no gain in simplicity*. Second, no one of the indices involves all three measurements, so *no one of them unifies the information*. Third, since any one of the indices can be expressed as a simple function of the other two, *one of the indices must be redundant*. Fourth, to deal exclusively with the indices involves *loss of information;* for one can show algebraically that while the indices can be calculated unambiguously from the measurements, the converse is not true. Given the three indices, one cannot find out what R, P, and H are. What has happened is shown in figure 11.1. The points that originally occupied three

---

*If, as it implies, the term *the percentage of normal prothrombin level* tells us accurately the proportion by which the function of the liver—the source of prothrombin—is depressed, that is another matter. But it is not at all obvious that this claim is true of percentage of normal prothrombin; or if it were, that it would bear any exact relationship to prognosis.

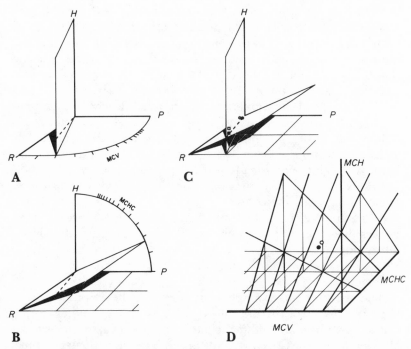

Figure 11.1. In diagrams *A*, *B*, and *C*, the three axes represent hemoglobin (*H*), red cell volume (*R*), and hematocrit (*P*); in diagram *D*, they are the mean cell volume (*MCV*), mean cell hemoglobin concentration (*MCHC*), and mean cell hemoglobin (*MCH*). *MCH*, the product of *MCV* and *MCHC*, occupies a single surface only (represented by the heavier grid lines). In *A*, all points on the particular surface shown have the same *MCV*. In *B*, all points on the surface shown have the same *MCHC*. In *C*, the two surfaces are shown as intersecting at the dashed line (which for reference is shown in *A* and *B* also). All points on this line have the same *MCV* and *MCHC* and therefore the same *MCH* also; they are marked by the same (black) point on the surface in *D*. There are two important consequences. First, given the latter point in *D*, one cannot uniquely identify where it came from in the *ABC* spaces, which implies loss of information. Second, the two square values in *C* are close and, therefore (one might expect), have similar meanings. The same is true for the black and white circular values. In contrast, one would expect the two circular points to have meanings very different from the two distant square points. But in *D* the two black symbols occupy the same site, and the two white symbols a different one. Spatial clusters in *D* do not mean the same as those in the other diagrams. Neither consequence is obviously absurd; but they are both disturbing.

dimensions (fig. 11.1A–C) now all fit on one plane (fig. 11.1D). But plotting them in the latter diagram requires either three pieces of information or any two of them together with either some non-trivial calculation or accurate drawing of a projection of a system with three dimensions in a two-dimensional diagram.

There are several lessons here. First, making effective indices from natural measurements needs some knowledge of how it should be done and what properties should be expected from such indices. Second, all the component readings are liable to some statistical variation, and then the indices may not be independent, a fact that may complicate interpretation. Thus, both *MCH* and *MCHC* have *H* in the numerator, so they are clearly not independent; besides, if through technical error *H* is underestimated, both indices will tend to be low, as a result of exactly the same error. Third, one wonders what may be gained? Economy is an attraction, but it is certainly not a feature of the present example. The clinician must now keep six sets of values in mind instead of three. Some scholarly hematologists with whom I have discussed indices say that they get no help from them. However, failure of these indices does not mean that one could not arrange the data more informatively.

Comment

The intent of this example is not to judge the empirical use of these indices. (Still less does it preempt what might otherwise be learned about them. Automatic particle counters allow *MCV* to be independently measured, for instance.) The analysis deals solely with the logical consequences of deducing these indices *from the same three data values* of *R*, *P*, and *H*. After the foregoing was written, a brief, penetrating paper by Fischer and Fischer (98), dealing with the same topic from an empirical standpoint, showed that *MCHC* is nearly invariant and quite uncorrelated with *MCV*. The low *MCHC* traditionally ascribed to iron-deficiency anemia is factitious.

Likewise, the statistician may go through his own operations, flawless by his professional standards, yet they may be just as wrongheaded as in the last two examples. Kimball (99) called one common blunder an error of the third kind, finding the right answer to the wrong question. The fault is no reproach to the statistician's professional skill. The mathematical statistician or the clinician may not be equipped by training to understand or to answer a question in French; and while the glib solution is to seek the aid of an interpreter, even expert interpreters may miss professional subtleties.

Example 11.14. To take a facetious, but not a trivial, example, a physician examining a patient's chest with pneumonia or pleurisy in mind will ask the patient to say "ninety-nine," a phrase chosen, not on its mathematical merits, but because its telltale resonances may be distorted by either of these diseases in a characteristic fashion. If the patient is French, the interpreter (if well informed medically) will not ask the patient to say "quatre-vingt-dix-neuf," but "trente-trois" (33); and the physician interpreting any distortion in what he hears must know what this French phrase sounds like in a normal chest. It has its own resonances, which differ from the English translation.

Now comparable pitfalls can arise in statistics; and while one may hope that alert and interested statisticians will take the trouble to get the context of the question clear, there is nothing in their training that requires them to be able to do so. The result may be that the problem the biologist wants to solve and the answer that the statistician provides may have very little to do with each other. This breakdown does little harm when it irritates the scientist, because he will reject it. The real danger is that neither the biologist nor the statistician may realize that any breakdown has occurred. Like the interchange between the two deaf gentlemen in the park,* it may create that ultimate devastation of the intellect: an illusion of understanding.

The Development of a Model

It is a concern of the biomathematician to respect at once both the mathematical soundness of his model and its biological relevancy. But that way of putting it may mislead somewhat. It is not necessary, indeed it is scarcely practicable, for both facets to be addressed completely and perfectly at the same time. A common technique for apposing them is that known as *iteration,* that is, guessing at the answer, seeing how well it fits, adjusting it to improve the accuracy of the second guess, and so on.

Example 11.15. Purely as an analogy, suppose we are required to solve the equation $y = x^5 + x = 20$. Now theory shows that this particular equation is one of those that cannot be solved by systematic algebra; yet when a geneticist or a physiologist is faced with such an equation, he has no choice but to solve it, using some kind of iteration, a sort of systematic trial and error. One such attack is shown in table 11.1. Initial guesses that x is 1 and that it is 2 give values for y (the left-hand side of the equation) that are too low and too high respectively; that is, they *bracket* the solution. There are various ways of iterating. A simple one we shall use here is to guess some intermediate value between the closest bracketing values so

---

*"Is this Wembley?" "No, Thursday." "So am I. Let's go and have a drink!"

Table 11.1. Solution of an Equation by Simple Iteration

x	$y = x^5 + x$	Desired value for y
1	$1 + 1 = 2$	20
2	$32 + 2 = 34$	
1.7	$14.2 + 1.7 = 15.9$	
1.8	$18.9 + 1.8 = 20.7$	
1.79	$18.377 + 1.79 = 20.167$	
1.786	$18.17219 + 1.786 = 19.95819$	
1.787	$18.22312 + 1.787 = 20.01012$	
1.7868	$18.21293 + 1.7868 = 19.99973$	
1.78691	$18.218533 + 1.78691 = 20.005443$	
1.786806	$18.2132316 + 1.786806 = 20.00003762$	

far available. One might guess that the solution is closer to 2 than to 1 and try 1.7. At this value, the answer is closer, but still too low. On the other hand, 1.8 is a little too high. We may push the search as far as accuracy requires. There are *systematic,* and more efficient, patterns of making the adjustments than this simple guessing, but the broad idea of iteration will be clear enough.

A biomathematician may set out with high hopes for a particular model, but will be wise not to expect it to fit the facts exactly. He should be prepared to make some adjustments in the values he gives his parameters or even, if necessary, in the detailed structure of the model. In the analogy, we may regard the model as the first guess at the answer and the predictions from it as being the counterpart of computing $y = (x^5 + x)$. Matching them against the empirical data is rather like matching y against 20 in example 11.15. If the match is not exact, then something may have to be modified in the model. However, if the match is a good one, the biomathematician will apply a more demanding test, just as, in table 11.1, we press the answer by carrying the calculations to more decimal places. And just as we will in time run out of significant figures on the calculator, the biomathematician may be unable to test his model beyond a certain point because the resolving power of the data he can obtain cannot be improved further. Newtonian physics, for instance, passed all empirical tests available until the late nineteenth century, when the resolving power of science had become fine enough to show that there were flaws. The lesson should be savored; for when Einstein replaced Newton, it was soon seen that a first-order approximation to Einstein's theory gives us back Newton's theory, which, for most practical purposes, can still be used as an adequate substitute. Thus, we may say that Einstein did not totally demolish Newton's analysis, but refined it, by showing that in special circumstances it must be fine-tuned.

Example 11.16. Everybody who has learned a little conventional geography will be familiar with the need to draw simplified maps. This art furnishes a nice analogy to what we are about in biological modeling. Too little attention to details of shape will be unworkably vague; too much will swamp the memory. We take as an example the mainland United States. At the one extreme, one might regard it as simply a rectangle (fig. 11.2A). This would be a perfect descriptor for the limits of two of the states (Wyoming, and immediately south of it, Colorado) shown hachured in the diagram. They have boundaries defined in meridians of longitude and parallels of latitude; but for the whole country, it would be inadequate. By analogy, giving the length and breadth is rather like quoting the mean and variance (which cannot be improved on as descriptors of Gaussian data, but are, in general, not enough). A less modest descriptor might be to represent the coastline by a series of curved segments (all capable of being drawn by a standard set of draughtsman's French curves) such as those shown in figure 11.2B and C. They illustrate how illation enters the process. The scientist may be struck by a similarity between the projections of Maine and Florida and surmise that the map is symmetrical about a horizontal axis (the dashed line in B), and beyond that use only four paired segments. Or he may abandon symmetry, allow much more elaborate specifications, and focus on particular areas of interest (fig. 11.2C, which uses twenty-two segments). In all three diagrams, the discrepancy between the original map and the model map is shown in black. Map A is simple and easily stored as a few digits, but shows a good deal of black. C is much more complicated, but still much simpler than the original coast, and the amount of black is impressively less. The choice among the three representations would depend on what detail is thought important. The farmer might be content with B or even A, but call for details about mountains (which have been totally ignored). Yachtsmen would have less interest in mountains, but would regard even my "true" coastline as grossly inadequate. To those interested in continental drift, C would certainly be good enough or even a little too detailed.

Example 11.17. Those concerned with patterns of skeletal growth know that people with long bodies have long legs, and conversely. As a gauge of proportions, it has been the practice (67) to use the ratio of u, the length of the upper body segment (from the crown of the head to the symphysis pubis), to w, that of the lower segment.

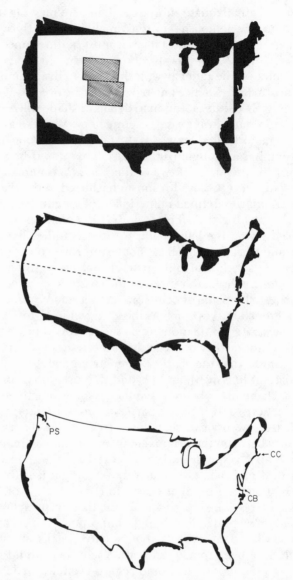

Figure 11.2. Descriptive geography of the land mass of the United States. In all three diagrams, a fairly detailed map is shown as a closed figure, and superimposed on it is another closed figure that is an approximation and has about the same area. The true coastline is used as the analogy of the truth; the fitted form is an analogy of the model. Discrepancies (that is, points that lie within one figure but not the other) are shown in black, and the smaller the amount of black, the better the fit. *A:* The model is rectangular. Shown as hachured shadows are the states of Wyoming (north) and Colorado (south), for which the rectangular model is perfectly apt.

Unfortunately, body proportions in children are different, the head being perhaps one-quarter of the total height, compared with one-eighth in an adult. In unpublished data we find that the distortion of using the adult ratio in a child may be almost entirely corrected by taking the index $u/(w + m)$, where m is a constant to be found empirically. One may then assess the body proportions *ignoring age altogether*.

This example illustrates the simplest kind of scientific iteration. Let us consider the steps a little more closely.

1. The issue is congruity, which is of some interest because when stature is disordered, it may be the legs that are shortened (for instance in achondroplasia) or lengthened (in the Marfan syndrome); the trunk may be shortened (in Morquio's disease, etc.); or both may be shortened, as in pituitary disease. The most elementary objective gauge is to deal in proportions, which suggests using ratios.

2. Looking at ratios certainly helps; for patients with the Marfan syndrome are certainly not all the same height, and the length of leg alone is not really a good discriminant. However, the ratio is by no means foolproof. For the kinds of ratios found in healthy people depend on age. The brain matures early, and it is hardly surprising therefore that its container, the skull, changes less than the trunk and limbs. So back to the drawing board.

3. Let us suppose that at birth the length of the upper segment has a certain ratio to that of the lower, and that both grow at a constant rate, but the rates differ for the two segments. Then it is not hard to show that by adding (or subtracting) an appropriate quantity to (or from) the lower segment, a fixed ratio of lengths will result.* This maneuver is equivalent to saying that if we graph the upper segment against the lower, regardless of

---

*Let u, the length of the upper segment, be a at birth, and grow b_1 each year, so that $u = a + b_1x$ at age x. Likewise, let the lower segment, w, be ca at birth, and grow at rate b_2, so that $w = ca + b_2x$. Write m for $-a(c - b_2/b_1)$. Then $u/(w + m) = b_1/b_2$, a constant.

B: The model is made symmetrical about the dashed line and is limited to the four paired segments of standard French curves. *C:* Symmetry is abandoned, and the number of segments increased to twenty-two. Particular attention is paid to Puget Sound (*PS*), Cape Cod (*CC*), and Chesapeake Bay (*CB*). The tension lies between simplicity (which decreases from above down) and fidelity (which increases from above down).

   age, a straight line will result *but* (*without an adjustment of the data*) *it will not go through the origin.*
4. We try this idea, and behold! it works. The adjusted ratio no longer seems to depend on age. Instead of constantly referring to McKusick's graph or memorizing separate sets of values for individual ages, the clinician now can get away with learning three quantities, namely, the value he must subtract, and the limits of the range of ratios in which he is interested.
5. Nevertheless, empirical success is not enough for the authentic biomathematician; one must also think about meaning. The scientist will wonder whether this new model for body proportions makes sense. Most immediately there are two objections.
   First, it is obvious that the length of neither segment goes on increasing in a straight line with age: it stops altogether in early adult life. True. But this objection is not so troublesome as it may first seem. We can imagine graphing the actual growth curves on an elastic sheet and stretching it unevenly in such a way as to make the curves into straight lines. To be sure, the scaling on the time (or age) axis will look rather odd (fig. 11.3); but that is neither here nor there, because the final goal is to find an index in which age may be ignored entirely; so it cannot ultimately matter what we do to the age scale. All that is necessary to defend the new index is that the old stretching of the time axis will apply *equally to the growth curves of the two body segments.* While this last assumption may not prove to be true in fact, the immediate theoretical objection has been demolished.
   The second objection is more formidable. Surely it is very naive to suppose that something so complicated as the upper segment (comprising such structures as the skull, neck, thorax, and abdomen) can usefully be represented not only by a simple growth formula but by one of the same (linear) form as the lower segment? Again, the former issue can be dealt with by the logical device of the elastic stretchable sheet; but the latter objection cannot be brushed aside because it is almost certainly true. There is no room for complacency at our success so far; there is undoubtedly need of further refinement. Even so, we should not belittle the improvement that has been achieved.

   Comment. What is a realistic assessment of our progress? First, the new index is at least as *accurate* as the old, and certainly more economical. All the criticisms that can be leveled against the new (and there are many) apply equally well to the old. Wise biologists are always cautious about accepting the fidelity of some simple index to the biological details. But the issue here is not whether to

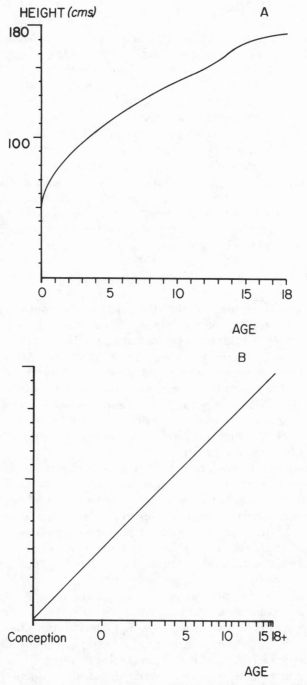

Figure 11.3. *A:* Schematic representation of how the height increases with age. *B:* The age axis has been transformed so that the growth curve is linear, which means that all ages beyond the final sealing off of the growing points of the bones (at about eighteen) are telescoped into one point.

accept the new test uncritically; it is how the new test compares with the old one. The comparison can be fairly made by using the same criteria for both. Second, however primitive, the new index at least begins to throw a little light on how and why the relationship changes with age; it is no longer a "black-box" descriptor. Third, in refining matters further, we have a good idea how and where to amplify and explicate. Thus, the new index has a *heuristic* value—rudimentary indeed, but a considerable advance. Fourth, from the statistician's viewpoint, this new treatment is an improvement. For one thing he no longer has to make the particular hidden assumption that error of measurement is strictly proportional to the true value (which does not at all seem a plausible assumption for height, though it might be for other measurements). Fifth, instead of grappling separately with comparatively small samples in a great many age groups—each of which he must treat without regard to the others—by eliminating the effect of age, he is able to pool all the results.

Nevertheless, the fact that the analysis represents a clear advance must not be taken to mean that the matter is now finished. Even if (which I doubt) it proved to be the last word on the relationship of the upper body segment to the lower, we must recognize that these measurements are, at best, coarse and far removed from the site at which the gene acts. One could marshal reasonable arguments that growth of the femur and that of the tibia are under separate genetic control (as is evident from the varied degrees to which they are affected by various genetic disorders) and that they should be treated separately.

However, while this example is neither profound nor intricate, it does show something of the twin concerns of authentic biomathematical modeling. It has allegiance to biology and to mathematics. It is concerned with enriching meaning in both spheres. It is fostering the union; it shows both how the mathematical reasoning might develop and what further (and perhaps more illuminating) data might be collected. It has promoted generalization (pushing a principle beyond age) and might readily do more. Some similar minor adjustment might provide an index that would apply to all racial groups or even to different animal species. Finally, by its enquiring tone, it is directing attention to components and mechanisms and away from the soporific seduction of descriptive statistics.

Example 11.18. An admirable example of authentic biomathematical modeling is Knudson's analysis of the genetics of retinoblastoma (65). In the development of the retina, an embryonic cell called the retinoblast matures into the adult form. While immature, it may develop into a retinoblastoma, a cancer encountered in childhood only. Now it is clear from Macklin (100) and from other writers that this tumor may run in families; but the details of inheritance are puzzling, despite cosmetic appeals to a structureless entity called "incomplete penetrance" to cover up the blemishes. Roughly, the data show that the family clustering is strongest among those in whom the disorder affects both eyes; that the concordance rate in identical twins is higher than in nonidentical, but never attains 100 percent; and that no matter how strong the hereditary pattern, not always are both eyes of a person affected. How is all this to be accounted for?

One extreme approach is to look at the issues from a statistical point of view: to describe, not to explain or (in a narrow sense) to account for the discrepancies from Mendelian theory. One might compute empiric risks as Macklin did (100). One might find out whether multiple retinoblastomas ever occur in the same eye, and if so, how the numbers are distributed. One might look at the distribution of the age of onset or diagnosis. As we shall see later, these approaches have their merits. In the terms of chapter 8, they address etiology rather than pathogenesis.

The other extreme is to focus on more and more detailed studies of the retinal cell, to try to find animal analogues, and the like. To isolate an abnormality—a defective enzyme or a chromosomal disruption—would lend zest to the chase. It would certainly give us a flying start in the understanding of pathogenesis. But there are snags in this approach. First, plausibility. A *simple* enzyme defect could hardly explain the bizarre pattern of inheritance. Second, focus. The narrow scientist does not really know what he is looking for; so there is no assurance that he would see the defect even if it were staring him in the face.* Third, formality. The mere fact of finding an abnormality would neither capitalize on nor refine the empirical data on the peculiar risks of being affected. I see no hint that the precision of genetic counseling (other than antenatal diagnosis by amniocentesis) would improve: to the contrary, such a discovery (if one is to judge by many analogous instances) would lead most human geneticists, even many clinical ones, to argue that

---

*Ramon y Cajal (101) seems to have noted the variable presence of a compact mass of chromatin in certain tissues. The fact that it was present in normal women but not men was first noted in 1950 by Barr et al. (102). In contrast, surmise anticipated observation in the analyses by Waardenburg (103) and Bleyer (104) suggesting that Down's syndrome is a chromosomal anomaly. It took twenty-seven years to find it (78).

the questions should be asked and answered in terms of the underlying anomaly and that the clinical picture is too crude to engage their attention. (Witness the almost total lack of concern with the age of onset and the clinical course of a disease once its etiology is discovered.)

Knudson saw the perils of both extremes and set out to capitalize on what could be learnt from the facts. First, a tumor suggests some kind of a radical change in the cell, and it is likely to be a random one, since not all those at risk develop it. One possibility is that the insult is environmental, and one thinks of mutagens. But even under heavy provocation, mutations are excessively rare events, occurring with a probability of perhaps one in ten-thousand to one in a million. What could offset this implausibly low risk? One clear answer is a large number of cells that are each at some such low risk. If there are five million retinoblasts (a figure that is approximately correct) at a risk of one in a million, on average, five will be affected. But if so, why is the risk not high in everybody? Knudson's surmise is that in the inherited cases, the cells at birth are not affected, but are already vulnerable: for instance, there may normally be a fail-safe or repair process that in familial retinoblastoma is inherited in damaged form, and a single further insult may suffice to cause a tumor. The details of the possibilities are many. A least-complicated model is shown in figure 11.4. The calculations are merely illustrative, not exact; but they could be adapted to fit the data. Those at "inherited" risk carry the abnormality (represented by the half-black symbols) at all stages—as a zygote and then in all the cells of both eyes. Between birth and full maturation, some stimulus such as a certain kind of light wave completes the damage, and the tumor results; and since there are millions of cells in the retina, the risk will be high and equal, perhaps independent, in the other eye. Those without the inherited risk require two insults *in the same cell,* which makes the condition very unlikely; and the risk of this double event happening in both eyes is negligible.

Now the idea of a disease being caused by a succession of insults was not novel (63, 105, 106); nor is the idea of an environmental insult causing cancer (107). But the richness in Knudson's model is that, first, it can be adapted (by estimation) to fit the facts. Second, one idea is explaining several facts: why, for instance, the tumor is not present in all at risk; why when it is present it is not always bilateral; why bilateral tumors almost never occur in the non-hereditary type; why multiple tumors virtually never occur in one eye except in the inherited cases. Third, it leads to particular predictions that can put it to the test: for instance, what the risk should

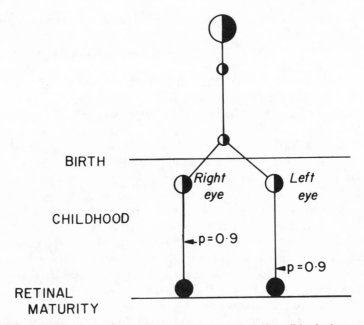

Figure 11.4. Knudson's model. Retinoblastoma develops if a cell in the immature retina receives two (photic) insults. In the "hereditary" type (shown here), one insult is built into the genotype, and only one more insult is needed in any cell between birth and retinal maturity to produce the tumor. Since there are some five million susceptible cells, the risk of at least one being hit is fairly high; and while it is not certain, there is a high probability that it will occur in both eyes. In the nonhereditary type, the risk of a cell being hit once may be much the same, but the probability of that same cell being hit again is very small. Children that do not have the first insult built in greatly outnumber those that do. However, a double hit in them is a rare event compared with a single hit in the hereditary type. These probabilities balance out, and the hereditary types will not be conspicuously commoner in ascertained children. However, the probability of both eyes being affected will be minute in the nonhereditary type. For the same reason, multiply affected members in a family will be far more common in those with the built-in first insult, although even in identical twins one will not expect a concordance rate of 100 percent.

be in relatives of probands with unilateral and bilateral tumors respectively and what the ratio of the risks of the two types should be; how the time of diagnosis should be distributed (granted a one-hit process); and what the distribution of the number of separate tumors in one eye should be and the times between their appearances. Fourth (whether it proves true or not), there is authentic biological content in the model. It lends shape to the appropriate course of empirical investigation. The biologist now works on the supposition that he has two steps to discover, and the attendant risks appear to be very different. Fifth, it raises fundamental questions that would not otherwise have been apparent as to the dynamics of the defect, what its risk and rate of dying out would be. Sixth, it paves the way for the analysis of other, more complicated tumors. Knudson does not have it all his own way; and the critical review by Matsunaga is worth consulting (108).

Example 11.19. As a last example of modeling in Medicine, let us consider homeostasis. In chapter 7 we considered some features of the balancing process that depends on feedback. We saw that if the restoration process is vigorous enough, it will overshoot and lead to a damped, a steady, or even an amplifying tremor. But the response does not depend on the *scale* of the upset. If the disturbance is made twice as large, every stage of the process will be made twice as large; but whether or not it overshoots and (if it does) how it oscillates with time in no way depend on the size of the displacement. By this kind of model one can explain reasonably well many phenomena such as tremors, reactive hypoglycemia, Cheyne-Stokes respiration. However, it asks the scientist to believe certain things that are not always plausible: for example, that the vigor of response of the processes by which the standing position is maintained are proportional to the degree by which it was disturbed.

Now that relationship may be true up to a point; but it will inevitably break down at extremes: tripping over an object or a forceful movement, such as a blow or a body charge at football. If this simple model were literally true, the person could never be knocked off his feet; and while the objection to this absurdity might be countered by saying that the homeostatic effect is being contaminated by the effect of inertia, there are many other instances (such as exposure to extreme cold) in which no inertia is involved, and yet the more extreme perturbations may be too much for the body to overcome. The scale of the disturbance *is* important, and if the model proves otherwise, then we should wonder how to reconcile the differences. One might, for instance, wonder whether the issue is one of homeostasis at all. (It seems doubtful, for instance, that heat stroke is simply overloading of the cooling process.) But also we might raise the question of whether the restorative force is more than a simple proportionate one; perhaps it depends on the size of the displacement raised to some power, in which case the scale of the displacement could no longer be ignored. Or conversely, it may be that small displacements are not adjusted at all. One might plausibly argue that the balancing skill of the acrobat depends on detecting, and at once righting, minute displacements that most people would not detect, or would respond to more slowly. But neglected drift is not the only cause of imbalance; the corrective process may be overzealous. This example could be end-lessly elaborated. But the fact that the complexity of the process might be more subtle than at first supposed, or that the complexity differs according to the process concerned, must not exact the risk that in the first brush with the problem, the scientist become so bogged down with possible complexities that he never gets started at all.

Commentary
This last fact merits a broad cautionary comment. The two extreme approaches—vagueness to the point of chaos at the one end and excessive structuring at the other—are equally harmful to understanding, though for quite different reasons. Vagueness means that there is no cutting edge to the idea at all: nothing can be verified or falsified, and the conclusions will be so vaporous as to be of no help scientifically or clinically.

A model that has too much detail may be equally futile for two reasons. One defect is that if there are too many unknowns in the equation, it may be extremely difficult to get even rough estimates of any of them. The other is rather more difficult to put into words. Generally, a heavily structured model tends to have corporate effects that have less and less to do with the components. As we saw in chapter 4, under very broad assumptions, the sum of a great many random variables will tend to follow the Gaussian distribution (q.v.), regardless of the characteristics of the component parts. This property is widely used in statistical practice and makes many difficult problems easy to handle, at least approximately. But we get nothing for nothing. This admirable principle about many added effects ("the central limit theorem") means that if we have nothing but a Gaussian variable, it is a thankless task to find what kind of a system it came from, for a great many systems will be rendered indistinguishable by it. It is a little bit like a tracker examining a road that has been walked on by many people. It is easy for him to recognize that many people have walked on it, but difficult to identify all the individual footprints. Thus emerges the clash that we have stressed throughout this chapter: that between the statistician's drive to describe and the biologist's drive to unravel. They really are antithetical: the easier the task is for one, the harder it is likely to be for the other. The biologist's search is made easier by the obstinate preservation of the features of every part; the statistician's is made easier by an anonymous character in the individual components. This conflict of demands leads to the estrangement between the molecular geneticist and the classical quantitative geneticist; or the student of populations and the clinician; or the humanistic cult of the individual and the engineer's appeal to statistical mechanics.

When I say that there is a clash, I would not have it understood in any polemical sense. Obviously, both kinds of information have their uses that should be seen as complementary rather than competitive. Nevertheless, this difference in focus has often led to an unfortunate breakdown in communication among proponents of the two kinds of approaches.

PROBLEMS

11.1. How would you refute *rigorously* (that is, not by rhetoric or by woolly arguments) the claims of those who believe:
   a. The world is flat?
   b. The blood does not circulate, but ebbs and flows?
   c. Base metals may be turned into gold?
(The value of this exercise would be greatly enhanced by having a debate in which one side tries its hardest to defend the claims seriously and to undermine the arguments of the opposite side. The onlookers would benefit most from voting *fairly according to the honest merits of the arguments advanced* and not on the views that they have come to hold as a result of cultural indoctrination.)

11.2. What would you guess the following Spanish medical words mean: *angina, constipado, erupto, afonica?* When you have answered, find out what they do in fact mean.

11.3. Verify the formula given in the note to example 11.17 and work out a numerical example. Find an intuitive explanation for why proportionality has been restored by adding (or subtracting, as the case may be) an appropriate constant to one or the other of the measurements. (Hint: Draw a graph of the results.)

11.4. Investigate the advantages, defects, and pitfalls of the use of ratios.

11.5. "It takes multiple components (words, figures, ink particles, etc.) to record one datum. Therefore, to represent all the facts about all the particles in the universe would require more components than there are particles. Therefore, all the facts in the universe can never be recorded, even in principle. Therefore, we can never verify any universal. Therefore, scientific knowledge cannot exist." Comments?

11.6. Should dentists be able to extract square roots?

12 | Disease, Classification, and Normality

Once more we return to the issue of grouping. In chapter 8 we dealt with this problem and its various implications. But the approach there was theoretical, even austerely so. There the questions were: Why should diseased states be seen in terms of classes? What are the ultimate realities of disease, realities that do not depend on arbitration? What can we learn from looking more and more closely at association among traits, at pathogenesis, at etiology? Here we take a much more utilitarian view. We are still asking *why?* but the focus is on motives for classifying rather than on reasons for doing so.

After thinking and writing about this problem for many years (11, 91, 109), I conclude that my own profound puzzlement over the problem stems largely from the elusive and gratuitous assumption that the problem to be solved is universal, unique, and homogeneous. It is only too easy to start from one rather crass viewpoint and go on to dangerous generalizations.

Consider some gross congenital defect—say, a fetus born without a head. We might then argue that it is a flagrant abnormality: not by the most sardonic stretch of the imagination is it a mere exaggeration of a tendency present in all of us; and we go on to argue that disease is clearly something apart from health, that we must keep this idea clearly in mind even if from time to time the distinction may prove a little fuzzy.

It is just as easy (and as misleading) to say that everything one sees in the psychotic is present to some degree in all of us; that a person with high blood pressure is just like a person with low blood pressure except that his blood pressure is higher; that *disfigurement* is merely a sonorous French name we use to excite compassion, whereas its Nordic counterpart, *ugliness,* is used to express abhorrence, even hatred*; that too much fuss has been made about the difference between the social drinker (one that drinks less than we do) and the alcoholic (one that drinks more), the distinction being (appropriately enough) on a sliding scale. It tells us more about the doctor than about the patient. And from this second starting point it is tempting to suppose that the diseased is only quantitatively different from the normal, not qualitatively.

SOME KEY ISSUES

Diversity of the Questions about Diseases

In problems such as this, where there are arguments on both sides (that, taken one at a time, are hard to gainsay), it is a wise precaution to look into the possibility that the question being asked is heterogeneous and therefore does not admit of one homogeneous answer. In the same fashion many broad views of Things In General have had a certain truth and an area of sound application. Yet time after time these useful perceptions have been brought into disrepute by those who attempted to deal with all conceivable topics of discourse within the same analytical framework.

Example 12.1. The idea of the essence of a sphere—that set of criteria by which we put an object under the heading *sphere*—makes very good sense. The sphere is a useful mathematical notion that has changed little in thousands of years.

Example 12.2. To suppose that the notion of essence can be applied equally well to a cloud seems to me much more doubtful. The idea of a cloud is indeed cloudy: a vague sensory impression that has been radically revised since we have gone from painting pictures of it to flying through it.

Example 12.3. To use the term *essence* of colors (in the face of what physicists and physiologists now know about the topic) seems ludicrous. A color as a totally distinct thing is an idea that scarcely anybody but a child can now take seriously, as can be easily verified by observing a lexicographer squirming over the definition of *red,* or by noting that a dress designer or a manufacturer of paint has a huge list of qualifiers of colors, without which they could not market their wares; and not merely can one construct an unbroken gradation of color from one end of the visible spectrum to the other but, since Newton, it has been established that there is a

*It is interesting that the German word *hässlich,* means both "ugly" and "hateful."

precise correspondence between the gradation and the physical properties (notably the refraction) of light.

So it might be wise not to approach the topic of this chapter with narrow concerns about who is going to win, and by how much. The sensible clinician will want to judge each case on its merits; and the criterion most to hand will be not so much how much chopping up can be done as how much impact it has in a clinical context.

Let us start off with the idea that there is probably something to be said for both views, and perhaps others, and to see what we can learn from the appropriate examples that could be advanced.

A great deal of the difficulty about the merits of the problem arise from a failure to grapple with the origins of the existing confusion. For the time being let us suppose that there really are things in the domain of reality that are compact and distinct.

Example 12.4. We do not find it too hard to believe that hydrogen atoms differ radically from oxygen atoms; that (setting aside isotopes) hydrogen atoms are indistinguishable one from another; and that oxygen atoms are also. If those notions can be accepted, when they are dealt with one at a time, any variation among members of a group must be errors of observation, measurement, sorting. The variations within groups may tell us some home truths about current scientific methods; but they do not really tell us anything about the atoms. The natural and reasonable course, then, is to classify the atoms as best we can, blush at our mistakes, but dismiss the errors of misclassification as annoying but not in themselves informative. The sooner we can rid ourselves of errors, the better. So far, so good.

However, do all problems have the same structure? With sufficiently deep insight into what is being studied, it might be possible to end up by following the same pattern: that the information could be sorted into the things that matter and the things that do not. We would hence simplify the task of interpreting the data. In Medicine, one touchstone against which to test this question is prognosis. Consider three examples.

Example 12.5. It may be that some measurement is important only insofar as it points to a diagnosis. The rate at which red cells settle out of standing blood (the erythrocyte sedimentation rate, or ESR) is one such test. It is speeded up in a number of diseases, such as cancers of various types. To my knowledge, the ESR is of no importance in itself. If somebody were to discover a way that would restore a high ESR to normal but had no effect on the underlying cancer, I do not fancy that any clinician would have the slightest interest in using it, any more than a radiotherapist seeing the shadow produced on an X-ray by pneumonia would propose to treat it by taking a more penetrating X-ray. However imperfectly the underlying disease is understood or defined, in such cases the finding (the ESR or the chest X-ray) is, as it were, not in itself part of the prognosis, merely evidence with a bearing on it.

At the other extreme, there are disorders in which the measurement is the very channel through which the prognosis is expressed, the point of the point.

Example 12.6. The overwhelming prognostic significance of the diagnosis of migraine is that it produces headaches. To my knowledge the disorder has no other importance, although rarely it may perhaps lead to paralysis or other disorders of the cranial nerves. The efficacy of treatment is judged solely and precisely by whether the headaches occur and, if so, how often and how severely.

Example 12.7. There are other disorders in which the measurement is both a diagnostic feature and part of the prognosis in its own right. For instance, one of the features of chronic nephritis (of various types) is that the blood pressure is high. This sign is not very specific, since there are many other diseases that cause it. However, given that the diagnosis has been made, the blood pressure tells the clinician something about the stage that the disease has reached. In this sense, the blood pressure is a prognostic sign. But also, the level of blood pressure is important in itself: it increases the burden of work on the heart; it produces retinal change that, if neglected, may lead to blindness; it increases the risk of cerebrovascular accidents. These major contributory causes of disability and death are all much improved by lowering the blood pressure, although doing so does not abolish or reverse the original damage to the kidney.

As to prognosis in these three groups, it is clear that our attitudes may, and should, vary widely as to how far the prognostic feature is to the point. We might argue that if there were a foolproof method of diagnosing and assessing the severity of the cancer (or whatever the underlying condition may be), nobody would bother to measure the ESR; for the latter sign is a "noisy" one: the information in it is smudged by the effects of many factors that have little to do with the cancer (in which the clinician's real interest may lie). The exact opposite is true of the migraine, in which it would be quite meaningless to try to separate the signs and the prognosis. One could make nothing whatsoever of the statement "The patient's sick headaches are much worse than he thinks they are"; or "Although the patient is eight feet tall, he need not worry about bumping his head as he goes through doorways, because the X-rays of his skeleton show that he is suffering from a form of dwarfism."

Objectives of Elucidating Disease

It will perhaps be clear that we are not trying to solve the same question in every case. But also we are not necessarily trying to find the same answer. How the clinician looks on, or classifies, a disease depends on whether his motive for doing so is treatment, prognosis, collection of vital statistics, understanding basic mechanisms, the inheritance, the prevention. These aspects are all important; but they have different methodologies and different criteria. What may be an exquisite concern in one field may be a trivial elaboration in the other. It is possible that all can be dealt with in the same ultimate terms, and it would certainly be both helpful and reassuring if they could. But we are not entitled to demand that they should, nor do we expect that for those of us dealing with practical management of actual patients it would be convenient always to be dealing with ultimate terms.

Example 12.8. A famous example from physics was the rivalry between the corpuscular and the wave theories of light. Each seems to have its own area of aptness and utility. The firm conviction that the same quality, light, underlies both, has furnished the physicists with a formidable problem of reconciliation. Nevertheless, the cardinal problem does not have to be solved in order to equip a presbyopic patient with a helpful pair of reading glasses.

One can think of plenty of instances of clearly distinguishable states that have no prognostic implications, and conversely. There is here a contrast, even a clash, between the questions "What exactly underlies the disorder?" and "What difference would it make if we knew?"

An Analogy of the Source of Disease

As an attack on the problem, let us consider an extended analogy between politics and genetics that I have developed elsewhere (47). It involves a good deal of stereotypy that I shall tone down later; but it will do as a first, rough approximation. The patterns are in common use.

The Monarchical Model. I mean by this term the system in which there is one factor that (*a*) is either present or absent and (*b*) makes an overwhelming difference to what happens.

Neither of these two properties is absolute.

Example 12.9. The classical instance is the Mendelian trait such as sickle-cell disease. A particular nucleotide change is present or not;

and the disruption it produces when present is striking. However, the severity is affected by other factors, notably the oxygen tension and the amount of circulating fetal hemoglobin.

Example 12.10. A somewhat looser example is the Down's syndrome, which is due to a supernumerary chromosome 21. While the typical pattern is clear enough, the disorder may be present to an extent that varies in two ways. First, only parts of the extra chromosome may be present (e.g., in a translocation). Second, the extra chromosome may be present in a variable proportion of the body cells (mosaicism).

Example 12.11. The role of a specific infectious agent in certain diseases would also be in the monarchical class. But it is not quite so pure. The organism is a necessary cause, but rarely a sufficient one: it must be present in circumstances in which it overwhelms, or at least taxes, the host sufficiently to produce overt disease.

It is doubtful that there is any disease (except for those that are at once fatal) that follows the pattern of the ideal monarchical model; but one may be prepared to accept this notion as at least an approximation, provided that one can unequivocally distinguish whether the factor is present or not.

The Feudal Model. This bears some resemblance to the foregoing, but the power (so to speak) is concentrated in several major areas instead of in only one. Needless to say, such a system would be harder to disentangle and is correspondingly difficult to illustrate. At the oligarchical end, it is not difficult to find disorders such as favism, or Knudson's retinoblastoma model (65), in which the disorder calls for the conjunction of two causes, one genetic and one environmental. In other instances, it may, perhaps, be necessary to demolish both of two mutually compensating mechanisms.

Example 12.12. Apparently there are in most people at least two genetic loci (i.e., four genes in all) that produce the alpha chains of hemoglobin. If one gene does not function, there is no detectable effect; if two, there is mild disability; if three, an anemia called major thalassemia; if four, fetal death occurs (110). Such a relationship, mutually supporting and compensating, is conveniently called a *parastasis* (11, 35).

Example 12.13. It can be more tentatively argued that atherosclerosis has a somewhat similar structure. There is no doubt that to an extraordinary and precocious degree it may be severally caused by disordered fat metabolism, by disorders that cause thrombosis, by local injury (such as jet lesions and narrowing of the aorta), and doubtless by other factors. All contribute in some degree, yet none is indispensible. It is tempting to wonder whether the results of these disturbances should be seen as different diseases. Yet they probably cannot be completely divorced from one another. No disorder of blood lipids, however severe, can explain why the lesions of atherosclerosis occur where they do; and the most ferocious disorder of coagulation could not readily explain the presence of lipids in the lesions.

The Proportional Democracy Model. Here, there is no sign of concentration of power. It is an anonymous assembly of many separate, independent, units, each with equal power; and the corporate effects are simply additive. Its components are anonymous in the sense that, should any one make a contribution to the total so conspicuous that its presence could be known or even suspected,* the assumptions underlying the model would be violated and its imputed properties demolished. The conditions underlying the model are precisely those of a free and secret plebiscite in which there is proportional representation and action. These are the very conditions that, for a large population, will give rise to the Gaussian (or "normal") distribution.

Example 12.14. The most famous example of this model is the theory of heritability due to Galton (111) and rationalized by Fisher (112). Some human traits (height, intelligence, blood pressure, blood cholesterol), and many traits of commercial value in livestock, have been analyzed in this fashion.

Whether this pure democratic model is apt for clinical purposes and whether it can be given a sound scientific standing are another matter. In principle, like any other model, it would be warranted by appeal to verifiability, falsifiability, its heuristic value, and all the rest. This kind of corroboration is hamstrung by two major problems in this case. First, the endless divisibility of the model—the endless supply of "interactions" that can be invoked to account for discrepancies between naive predictions and the observations— makes it difficult to imagine any circumstances in which this model could be shown to be unsound. Second, empirical corroboration (by finding explicit biological counterparts to the mathematical structures that are invoked in the model) imperil the fundamentally anonymous character of the model.

Example 12.15. Dahl and his associates (113, 114), by inbreeding rats, produced a strain that developed fatal hypertension when given dietary sodium in amounts harmless to most rats. Here is a

---

*Except by special means that have nothing to do with the phenotypic impact of the trait being studied.

nice example of genetic factors in a quantitative trait. However, later studies showed that most of the genetic contribution came from a single genetic locus. This outcome is a triumph of Mendelian genetics; but it has left the original democratic view in ruins; and clearly this will always be the result when the anonymity has been breached.

The Majoritarian Democracy Model. This pattern is one of "block voting": if some agreed proportion of the total is attained, a certain decision is carried out (in the United States ½ for election to office, ⅔ to override a presidential veto, ¾ to ratify a Constitutional amendment); otherwise, it is not. A miss is as good as a mile, and squeezing by is as good as a landslide. The voting is graduated, the outcome is all-or-none. The genetic counterpart (still a matter of surmise) is the so-called threshold model.

Example 12.16. A convincing case is made (115) that in normal formation of the palate, the two halves must reach each other and fuse by a critical stage of development, or pressure from the growing tongue will prevent them from joining; and then clefting of the palate will result. But this meeting does not have to be *precisely* timed. Some leeway exists, and should the halves grow faster than necessary and meet well before the deadline, no harm results. Like catching a train, there is a wide range of arrival times, but the result is simple: one catches the train or one misses it. It is plausibly surmised that the rate of growth is under the influence of many factors: many genetic, some nutritional, some hormonal, and perhaps others. The clinical outcome may not make the example perfectly apt; for there is an intermediate state known as submucous clefting, in which the mucous membrane is intact but there is nonunion of the bone beneath. Certainly, to the casual eye, a pattern results that may be readily enough mistaken for Mendelian, though closer scrutiny will show that the Mendelian segregation ratios are not correctly followed.

Example 12.17. A disorder in some ways more convincing is gout. Let us accept (naively, perhaps) that the cardinal failure is the precipitation as crystals of uric acid from solution in blood, which occurs at a critical concentration. Now the blood level of the latter may vary widely with something not unlike a Gaussian distribution. By all the foregoing arguments, we may be persuaded that many factors (some genetic, others environmental) control it, so that it is like the Galtonian system. But the expression is all-or-none; or, allowing for fluctuation in the actual blood level of uric acid, an intermittent all-or-none pattern.

These four illustrative models are nothing like an exhaustive catalogue even of the genetic issues. Cybernetic processes (or feed-back corrections) (41, 42, 58, 59, 73) are important and have properties quite alien to any of the foregoing. Fail-safe (35), epistatic (17, 35), and weakest-link (116) processes have odder properties still. My aim is, not to swamp the reader with detail, but rather to point out that there are a great many possible kinds of systems where there are multiple functioning parts. To say the least, it is a little ambitious to suppose that they should all fall in line with some shallow preconceived idea like a tidy classification of diseases.

Comment

It will be clear from the foregoing that we have two separate, but related, problems on our hands. The first is to distinguish between the noise and the message; the other is to discern the shape of the message. If I might indulge in yet another simile, it is rather like a cook preparing fruit and vegetables. The noise is like dirt, which is got rid of as quickly as possible. The shape of the washed fruit and vegetables will vary. Perhaps there are several distinct structures, not all reckoned to be of the same importance. The almond and the plum are roughly similar but are treated quite differently. In an almond, it is the kernel that we are interested in, and the soft overlying pulp is discarded (and indeed there is a familiar meta-phorical use of the word *kernel*). In the plum, the soft part is eaten, and the kernel is usually ignored. In the orange, the skin is peeled off. In the apple, it is debatable whether the skin is to be eaten or not. In an onion (another popular image), one may peel off layer after layer looking for the inner core and eventually realize that these very layers are the point; that there is no core. In the potato, there are not even layers. Now it would be difficult, if not frankly absurd, to propose one single set of universal instructions for a computer to prepare all conceivable kinds of fruit and vegetables regardless of type. Yet it seems to me that the shallower analyst tries not only to do the equivalent with data but also (so to speak) to include the dirt as part of the analysis. Common tendencies are: confusing variation with variance; failing to separate experimental error from the useful information; and the compulsion to work with balance sheets (so that every scrap of input, whether we know anything about it or not, must, by hook or by crook, be fitted under "genetics," "environment," or "interaction"). They have led to an almost total intellectual bankruptcy in certain areas of research.

Example 12.18. Suppose that an investigator wishes to find the specific radioactivity per milligram of a specimen of blood from a patient in the course of a study on red-cell survival. It is necessary to think of several components of measurement, including the following.

1. Random errors (due to minor slips in weighing, etc.), which are to be minimized by improving technique and that are not in any way useful.
2. Random error due to the probabilistic nature of radioactive decay. Biologically it is uninformative; but it does contain a message: the biophysicist uses it to check on electrical contamination (e.g., from the counting circuitry), by comparing the calculated with the observed random variation from radioactive decay.
3. A large, systematic, but message-free effect, the weight, when empty, of the container for the blood. (The weight of blood is found by differences.)
4. Any systematic variation in the blood itself (e.g., whether arterial or venous blood is used).
5. The message (here the proportion of labeled cells in circulation).

With this broad conceptual background, let us look at various ways in which we may explore the nature of disease.

CLASSIFICATION

To remove any technical ambiguity, I shall use the word *classification* to denote a process with two stages. First, one sorts out individuals into groups; second, one discards the evidence on which the first step was taken as having no further interest. Having established by a series of measurements that one patient has a disease, *A*, I have no further interest in the individual measurements. I am saying that the classification is a sufficient substitute for them.

Example 12.19. A woman either is or is not pregnant. When the question has been settled, the data are of no further interest. There are no degrees of pregnancy (though there may be degrees of uncertainty about whether it is present or not). However, discarding the data after the decision has been made is without prejudice to examining them or making further measurements in assessing how the pregnancy is faring.

With these ideas in mind, how, why, and when do we classify?

Conventional Wisdom

Classification satisfies a demand that appears to be either a natural tendency or a powerful cultural force, and if successful, one that leads, or that we think leads, to insight into the nature of things. The more successful it proves in the individual case, the more it sharpens the focus of enquiry and the easier it becomes to strengthen the classification.

Example 12.20. The chronic diseases of the lungs led to a dim recognition of the disorder "consumption," which was not at first clearly separated from what is now called chronic obstructive lung disease. Tissue pathology made the distinction clearer; and when the search for a bacterial cause was started, it was much more obvious where to look than it would have been without the tissue pathology. When Koch's bacillus (*M. Tuberculosis*) was discovered (56), it provided, so to speak, a new rallying point for the diagnosis, and it led to grouping together the Gohn focus (the primary infection in the lung) and the caseating lesions as aspects of one disease, while separating off sarcoidosis as a distinct disorder.

The reasoning in such a revolutionary process is intricate enough to merit a closer look. There are two goals. On the one hand, we are trying to find the cause of tuberculosis. On the other hand, we are trying to delimit what we are to call tuberculosis. They clash; and I doubt that both can be simultaneously resolved with irreproachable logic. If we had the disease defined beyond dispute, we could decide whether the bacillus is causative because, if so (for instance), the disease would never occur in its absence. But since the disease is *not* independently and indisputably defined, what are we to say if what appears to be the disease occurs in the absence of the organisms? Either it may mean that the disease has been mistakenly diagnosed or it may mean that the organism is not, in fact, the cause; or both may be true. Now Koch recognized these difficulties, and in a famous set of so-called postulates (they are really canons of proof), he pointed out the corroborative value of experimental studies in etiology as well. But at once we get into another loop of soggy logic. If the organism injected into an experimental animal does not produce tuberculosis, we may infer either that it is not the true cause or that the animal is immune; or both. The same kind of problem will apply to immunological criteria, and even to therapeutic criteria. None of these arguments would logically exclude the technical possibility that tuberculosis is due, not to *M. Tuberculosis*, but to a virus parasitic on it. (I am not putting that forward as a serious theory: I am arguing in principle. But the same kind of vulnerable logic led to mistakenly ascribing influenza to *H. Influenzae.*)

Example 12.21. This quandary leads us at once to see an ambiguity in the way we have used the idea of a "causative organism." In disorders such as malaria, the natural pattern of infection depends on both a microorganism (a protozoon) and an insect vector (*anopheles*). The fact that the pathologist can infect a patient artificially without using the vector (for instance by giving a direct injection of blood from an infected person) is interesting; but arguably it has nothing to do with the natural disease, any more than the effects of injecting pure staphylococcal endotoxin (if it were available) would warrant the claim that the common boil is not an infection but a chemical intoxication.

In these examples we perceive the danger of hasty manipulation of words as a means of understanding problems. Little good comes of trying to compress these complicated problems of dynamics, interaction, and criteriology into smooth statements about *A* being "the cause" of "the disease," *B*. The current state of our view of tuberculosis does not come from a single polarized local piece of logic but from a subtle integration of complex processes, values, and objectives. Since it is no easy matter to understand it, it would be foolish to suppose that the present view will never have to be modified. A better understanding of inflammation may in due course persuade us that sarcoidosis and tuberculosis are best seen as the same disease, triggered by different mechanisms. However, that view would have few supporters at present.

Simplicity
The variation in the appearances of some quantitative characteristic may be seen as comprising variation among groups and variation within groups. At times, the former is overwhelming and the latter negligible.

Example 12.22. The phenotypes for the major blood groups (wherever they can be measured) are of this kind. With competent testing there is little doubt whether a person is of blood groups A, B, AB, or O. What doubts there are arise almost entirely from technical errors. Very occasionally there may be genetic complications, e.g., concealment by the Bombay factor (117).

At times, the variation among members within a group cannot be totally ignored.

Example 12.23. For legal and social purposes, sex is a clear enough designation. This fact must not be obscured by the rare ambiguities that arise no matter what criterion of sex—anatomy, biochemistry, cytogenetics, physiology, or the immunological test for the Y antigen—be used. Nevertheless, it is arguable that the variation within members of the same sex is important from a psychological standpoint and perhaps from others.

However, a great many characteristics show little evidence of authentic grouping; and the main reasons are three. First, there may, in fact, be no nontrivial grouping (as would be true of the almost pure Galtonian traits such as obesity).

Second, what we can study may be so far removed from the basic cause that it is lost in accumulated noise.

Example 12.24. Penrose (118) gave a classical example in phenylketonuria, in which the grouping is unambiguous when one looks at the data on the blood level of phenylalanine, but is undetectable when hair color is used. Commonly it is supposed that the indefiniteness of the classification is due to the fact that one is too far from the business end of the problem. But that view involves the implicit assumption that the point of the point is the blood phenylalanine level and not the hair color. The view of the hairdresser would not be the same as that of the chemist as to which matters more. Most clinicians would probably think that the intelligence was the real point and that perfect control of blood phenylalanine is no consolation if the patient is severely retarded. But of course in practice the latter two outcomes are not competing with each other.

Third, there may be a well-defined cause that is operating in a graduated fashion.

Example 12.25. There is no doubt that lead taken by mouth is toxic; but the actual intake may vary widely, as may the clinical and biochemical findings. There is no level of intake that divides subjects sharply into those who are and those who are not intoxicated by it.

The Predicative Fallacy. One pitfall in logic is very common: the inference of grouping by the predicate. The fallacy is common in unconscious reasoning and the genesis of phobias. ("Tigers are dangerous. Tigers are striped. My carpet is striped. Therefore, my carpet is dangerous.") It is a common pattern of reasoning in schizophrenia (119). Only an insane or a primitive mind would consciously regard that as sound reasoning. But although scientists repudiate it, they do the same sort of thing all the time in "exercising their judgment" (i.e., guessing, not reasoning) about how to grapple with the unknown. Doubtless this habit of reasoning explains scientific fashions.

Example 12.26. A small, but secure, success in explaining high blood pressure by disease of the kidneys has led to much research to try to find more and more subtle kidney disorders in milder and milder hypertension. The reasoning is predicative: Nephritis causes changes in the kidney. Nephritis is associated with high blood pressure. Increasing age is associated with high blood pressure ("essential hypertension"). Therefore, increasing age is associated with changes in the kidney. The effort has been enormous; the tangible yield, slight. There comes a time at which one may conclude that there is something in this line of enquiry, but not much; and that one should be devoting substantial attention to other possible causes. The simplicity that the predicative fallacy prompts must be abandoned in favor of richer virtues.

CARDINALITY AND DIMENSIONALITY

If we are not to use classification, what other options are there? In grappling with that answer, we will do best, in the long run, to spend a little time with a simple but fundamental distinction. Consider the set of outcomes from a random process. We roll a die, and the outcome will be some number from one to six. Now we may ask two questions.

1. How many *possible* answers are there? Six. This number is termed *the cardinality of the set.*
2. How many *qualities* are represented in the outcome? One, the die number. This answer is called *the dimensionality of the sample space.*

Example 12.27. In my passport are recorded my year of birth, sex, weight, hair color, eye color, and race. The dimensionality is six. The cardinality (depending on the resolving power of the answers) might be a very large, even an infinite, number.

Example 12.28. Consider the blood cholesterol level. Its dimensionality is clearly one: Any particular outcome of it could be faithfully represented as a point on one axis of a graph. If the measurement is recorded to the nearest mg/dl, and if we allow a range of from 50 to 1,500 (or some such figures), the cardinality would be 1,451. Now the clinician may say that we should reduce this number to something more manageable: say, into the categories *low, normal, raised, high, very high.* What can be meant by saying that this arrangement is "more manageable?" It means, I think, that one can reasonably memorize details about five diagnostic categories, but not about 1,451 of them. But this statement raises the question of what would happen if one dealt with the reading itself and did not classify it at all. In what way is it more useful to tell us that Mrs. Brown's blood cholesterol is "in the very high group" than to say it is 1100 mg/dl? There is no single answer to that kind of question, because the answer depends on the implications. A few examples may help.

Example 12.29. Suppose that by technetium scanning in patients with lung cancers we conclude that one patient has no secondary tumors, one has only 1 of them, a third has 10, and a fourth, 317. It can be argued that the treatment for the first is local excision; that for the second, local excision of both the primary and the secondary tumors; and that beyond that, local excision should be followed up by chemotherapy—the precise number of multiple secondaries is neither here nor there. In effect, there are three useful classes, and from a therapeutic standpoint the cardinality is three. The implication is that the number of secondaries is not the real issue, but the fact that there is corroborative evidence of scattering helps us to represent the state of the patient.

Example 12.30. Consider the question of how much thiopentane should be given to a patient as an anesthetic. In general, the answer will depend on a number of factors (age, sex, metabolic rate, alcohol intake, idiosyncrasies, etc.). We might single out body weight. Granted that the larger the patient, the larger the dose, one could construct a more or less detailed table to show the relationship between weight and dosage. The cardinality would be as large as we could bother to make it; and the clinician would either have to carry the table around or memorize it. But the dimensionality is only two (dose and weight); and it may be that all that is needed is to remember one number—how many milligrams should be given per kilogram body weight.

Example 12.31. A physician who has to give a prognosis to a patient with high blood pressure may take several courses. He may make nothing but broad statements. He may look up, or recall, what the expectation of life for that level of blood pressure is. He may remember some simple formula relating survivorship to blood pressure. He may take the attitude that blood pressure has very little to do with prognosis except as it bears on the underlying disease.

If we apply this argument to example 12.28, we may suppose that low blood-cholesterol levels are associated with malabsorption, very high ones with myxedema, and so on; and that beyond telling us the diagnosis, the level is not to the point. If this view is correct, then we must wonder what purpose there can be in lowering blood cholesterol level in itself, as distinct from lowering it by changing the disease. Lowering the blood cholesterol in myxedema by treating the hormone deficiency is sensible, whereas lowering it by preventing absorption from the bowel is not.

It should be clear, then, that there are two related, but distinct, ways of grappling with disordered states.

1. By grouping into classes or categories
2. By argument from, and with, the critical measurements themselves

There may, in principle, be any number of groups; but if there is only one, containing all patients, it will not help to distinguish anything from anything else, even the sick from the healthy. If there are many categories, they will tax the clinician's memory, and the experience of any one category may be embarrassingly small. Finally, there may be no hint of grouping at all. In any of these three circumstances it is wise to consider abandoning classification altogether and to argue from the measurements themselves.

NORMALITY

When we talk about normality, we wake sleeping demons. One may vainly propose to give a simple arbitrary meaning to the word *normal* and by doing so to get around all the ambiguities; but it cannot be done. I have a list elsewhere—which is by no means exhaustive—of the various meanings of that word (11), ranging from abstract mathematical meanings at one extreme to deep moral judgments at the other. It is surprising how much confusion exists among them: how often, for instance, people suppose that a measurement in "normal people" (whatever they are) has a normal (i.e., Gaussian) distribution. It is an endless source of concern to me that people will say that the common cold is a disease responsible for so much loss of work each winter, and in the next sentence say that it is normal to have two or three colds each winter.

Doubtless, if we could define sharp edges on every disease, we would by subtraction find the normal. But many "diseases" are not, in their nature, unambiguously separable from the normal or from other diseases. I use the phrase *in their nature* advisedly; for I suspect that some people fancy that if only we knew enough about underlying mechanisms, we would find a pure crystalline disorder underlying every perturbation. Now whether that claim is true or not, time alone will tell. The main point I make is that we have no particular reason for supposing that it is invariably true; and there are a number of cases where the closer we look, the less likely that outcome seems; and the various genetic models discussed earlier suggest why.

In the light of what has gone before, we might wonder how normality and disease (its complement) are to be viewed. Is normality a class like "sphere" in example 12.1? If the Mendelian model were typical, this answer might be correct. It would not solve all our problems. If we are concerned with other traits, such as height or weight, the odds are that we cannot sustain the illusion of useful classes at all. Rather than talking about the normal, perhaps it would be more useful to think in terms of the optimal. And the optimal must be seen not only within the entire context of the person (proportion, symmetry, internal correcting mechanisms, interaction, cybernetics, and all the rest) but also in terms of the demands made by the environment.

PROBLEMS

12.1. In a study by Elsom et al. (120), physicians were asked to decide which of a set of weights, blood pressures, blood sugars, etc., fell within normal limits. It was found that the higher the physician's own values were, the more lenient his assessments were and the higher the limits of normality he set. Comment constructively on the implications of these findings for the classification of disease.

12.2. Consider the following prognosis. "The patient has a reasonable chance of getting better, but, of course, we are none of us going to live forever. Complications, should they occur, will make things worse. The disease commonly has a long course, but is often shorter. I speak in generalities, as I must. You can never tell in the individual case." Comments?

12.3. "It is unprofessional conduct to cause a disease in a patient. After birth, an opening (fistula) between the systemic and the pulmonary circuits is a disease. The Blalock-Taussig operation for the tetralogy of Fallot ("the blue baby syndrome") consists of making such a connection artificially. Therefore, the Blalock-Taussig operation is unprofessional." Comment on this argument, and explore what its implications may be for the definition of disease and normality.

12.4. Consider the following quotation from the distinguished theoretical physicist Sir Arthur Eddington (121): "Apart from deliberate use of the balance-sheet to conceal the situation it is not well adapted for exhibiting realities because the main function of the balance sheet is to balance and everything else has to be subordinated to that end" (p. 33).

12.5. In each of the following classes, which is the normal state, and why?
   a. Hemophilia or nonhemophilia
   b. Sickle hemoglobin or adult (A) hemoglobin

    c.   Rh positive or Rh negative

    d.   Right-handedness or left-handedness

    e.   A sterile colon or one containing *E. Coli*

    f.   Patency of the ductus arteriosus

12.6. There are four natural halogens: fluorine, chlorine, iodine, and bromine. In many places, the public health has been held to justify adding the first three to the diet, without explicit consent of the person; the first to prevent dental decay, the second to purify drinking water, the third to prevent a type of goiter once prevalent. Consider the issues involved in adding the fourth to reduce the incidence of crimes of violence.

Appendix:
Some Commonplace
Statistics

The aim here is not to furnish a brief course in statistical methods but to state briefly some of the more common methods that critical readers may wish to call on to check results in papers they may read. Needless to say, it is not possible to give any justification for these methods or why they are preferred. Having made bold to write this section, I might as well be hanged for a sheep as for a lamb. Many of the statements will be only roughly correct; and while I would stand behind them as at least approximately true, I do not suggest them as a gold standard. Those looking for more explicit methods such as are necessary to do research are advised to look elsewhere (122–24).

DESCRIPTIVE STATISTICS

It is difficult to think coherently about a large set of individual numbers; and the natural tendency is to seek some means of "boiling them down" to a few manageable figures. Sometimes it is easy to do so because we know the *form* of the variable as well as the specifications or *parameters*. A familiar analogy is the geometrical figure. If we know it is a circle, all that we need to know to draw the figure is the radius. If it is a rectangle, we need two specifications, the length and the breadth. More complicated figures require more specifications; and for some shapes it may be difficult to discern and describe any form. If so, we must fall back on a small repertoire of general devices, of which I shall mention a few.

The Range

In statistics, *the range* denotes the highest and lowest values a variable assumes. Where the true distribution is rectangular in form, that is the only information needed. In general, however, it does not tell us much. By and large, the more opportunities, the more extraordinary experiences one will have had. Thus, on average a large country is more likely to produce the most extraordinary members. The tallest man in the world is more likely to be Russian or American than Fijian. This fact is the source of the principal weakness of the sample range as a descriptive statistic: that it depends exquisitely on the size of the sample. Unlike the behavior of most statistics with increasing size of sample, the sample range does not tend to settle down to any final figure. If the range is small, it may be used as a guide. Should the range in a large sample be (say) 220 to 240 units, we are fairly confident that readings outside that range are fairly unlikely. But if the range is 70 to 800, we have little evidence for deciding whether readings of under 200 or more than 300 are at all common.

The Mode

Often used as a measure of the location of the values, the mode is that value that most commonly occurs in the sample. There may be two or more modes; the entire range may be a mode (as in the rectangular distribution in which all values are equally likely). If the measurements are beyond reproach, an assured mode may have useful descriptive value. But it is fragile. The observer may tend to favor certain values (e.g., to read blood pressures as multiples of 5); or there may be some oddity in a machine that tends to produce false clustering. Sample modes (except in very tightly controlled systems such as the chromosomes) tend to give rather unstable answers. Where discrete quantities are to be estimated, even among statisticians the mode may be the preferred statistic. No sane statistician would dispute that the appropriate estimate of the number of chromosomes per cell present in an unfamiliar species should be anything other than the sample mode. For the true answer must be a whole number; and while the mode is certain to be, the mean is not. An old-fashioned statistician analyzing a set of results by hand and, through human error, coming up with several answers for the same total would take, not the average, but the modal value.

The Median

It can be argued that the natural split in a population is that point at which half of the values lie below and half above. This point is known as the median or (reckoning by the proportion of values that are lower than it) the fiftieth percentile.

Percentile

Pediatricians are familiar with a more general set of such proportions. The third percentile of weight or height is that quantity that equals or exceeds 3 percent of values in the population.

By and large, the median and the percentiles are sound descriptors even if (for Mendelizing traits, for instance) they occasionally give anomalous results. They may be found from straightforward sample proportions after the sample values have been arranged in ascending order. But if the form of the distribution is known, it is usually possible to find more efficient ways of estimating them.

AVERAGES

The technique of finding the average is well enough known: one adds the quantities and divides the sum by the number of values. The sample average is always an accurate (i.e., unbiased) estimate of the true mean. Provided we do not tamper with the data (for instance by taking logarithms, square roots, reciprocals, or ratios), in the practical world we may always be assured that both the average and the true mean exist.

The sample average and the true mean have certain nice properties that are worth knowing something about.

1. They always have a value lying between the highest and lowest values. (This is a useful check on the soundness of the calculations.)
2. To find from data in inches what the average is in centimeters, we may either multiply each reading by the conversion factor (2.5400) and average, or average the results in inches and multiply by the conversion factor. In general, the average of a (a constant) times X is a times the average of X.
3. The average weight of a man and his clothes is the average weight of a man plus the average weight of his clothes. Formally, the average of $(X + Y)$ is the average of X plus the average of Y.
4. Extending points 2 and 3 and setting $a = 1/n$, we see that the average is always an accurate estimate of the mean, as we noted previously.

THE VARIANCE

We may take the average not only of a set of values but also of some processed version of them. If we denote the true mean of a population by μ, then for each value, X, we may calculate $(X - \mu)$

Table A.1. Estimation of the Sample Variance for the First Five Readings of Table 4.1

	x	$x - m$	$(x - m)^2$
	3.32	$3.32 - 3.604 = -0.284$	0.080656
	3.45	$3.45 - 3.604 = -0.154$	0.023716
	3.30	$3.30 - 3.604 = -0.304$	0.092416
	3.70	$3.70 - 3.604 = 0.096$	0.009216
	4.25	$4.25 - 3.604 = 0.646$	0.417316
Total	18.02	0.000	0.623320
Divide by	5		4
Mean	3.604		0.155830

Sample mean = 3.604
Sample variance = 0.155830
Sample standard deviation is $\sqrt{0.155830} = 0.395$

and square it. The average of this value is called the *variance*. It is always a positive quantity and measures how scattered the results are: a high value, as one might imagine, means a wide scatter. The square root of this quantity is the *standard deviation*.

In practice we rarely know μ and must make do with the sample average as an estimate of it, which we shall denote by M. The variance is now calculated in the same way as before, but if we want the estimator to be accurate, we divide the sum, not by the sample size, but by one less than it. An example is worked out in table A.1.

The variance and the standard deviation have the following properties.

1. The standard deviation is never greater than the range. This applies both to the true and the sample standard deviations. However, the *true* standard deviation may exceed the *sample* range.
2. Not all the sample data can lie either less than or more than one sample standard deviation from the sample mean. There is an analogous property for true values.
3. The standard deviation is in linear units, the variance in square units; and the same results apply as in ordinary arithmetic. We convert the standard deviation in inches into the standard deviation in centimeters by multiplying by 2.5400. We convert the variance in square inches into the variance in square centimeters by multiplying by $(2.5400)^2$. More generally,

$$\text{var}(aX) = a^2 \text{var}(X), \tag{1}$$

where a is any constant.
4. If X and Y are independent of each other—that is, quite unre-

Table A.2. The Short (and More Accurate) Way of Computing the Sample Variance in Table A.1

x	x^2
3.32	11.0224
3.45	11.9025
3.30	10.8900
3.70	13.6900
4.25	18.0625
Total 18.02	65.5674

$$\text{Sum of squares from mean} = 65.5674 - (18.02)^2/5$$
$$= 65.5674 - 64.944080$$
$$= 0.623320$$
$$\text{Variance} = 0.623320/4 = 0.15583^a$$

[a]This result is the same as given by the direct method in table A.1.

lated to each other in any way—then the variance of their sum is the sum of their variances. This principle can readily be extended to any number of variates. Thus, the variance of a sum of n independent variables each with the same variance, σ^2, is $n\sigma^2$. The variance of their mean (that is the sum divided by n or multiplied by $1/n$) is found, by applying formula 1, to be

$$\text{var}[(1/n)\text{sum}] = (1/n)^2 n\sigma^2 = \sigma^2/n. \tag{2}$$

Thus, the larger the sample, the smaller the variance of its average. When n is infinite, the average is zero and the sample mean is exactly equal to the true mean. This conclusion is a formal statement of the common belief that "there is safety in numbers."

5. Because the calculations shown in table A.1 are tedious, especially if the sample mean is an awkward number, a simple formula is to find the sum of the n data, which is here denoted by T, and the sum of the squares of the numbers (S) and find

$$W = S - T^2/n \tag{3}$$

W is exactly equal to the sum of squares of the deviations from the sample mean. As before, we estimate the variance by dividing by $(n - 1)$. The data of table A.1 are reworked in table A.2.

THE COVARIANCE

If in each of n members of a population we have data on two variables (as concrete instances, height and weight) we may com-

Table A.3. The Computation of the Sample Covariance

	x	y	$(x - m_X)(y - m_Y)$	
	−3.63	8.56	$[-3.63 - (-2.648)][8.56 - (-1.186)] =$	−9.570,572
	−4.81	4.95	$[-4.81 - (-2.648)][4.95 - (-1.186)]$	−13.266,032
	0.67	−5.44	etc.	−14.114,772
	4.50	−21.06		−142.059,352
	−7.66	5.00		−31.004,232
	−22.62	−6.65		109.127,008
	13.54	10.62		191.115,528
	−8.82	1.58		−17.071,752
	−2.52	−6.54		−0.685,312
	4.87	−2.88		−12.735,492
Sum	−26.48	−11.86		59.735,020
Mean	−2.648	−1.186		

Sample covariance = 59.735,020/(10 − 1) = 6.637

pute the sample mean and variance for each separately, as before. But we may also compute a new quantity, the covariance. We find the mean weight for all the subjects; then from the weight of the first subject, we take the mean; the deviation (with its sign carefully preserved) will be denoted by d_1. We do the same for each reading. Then we do the same for height, denoting the first difference by f_1, and so on. Of course, some of the deviations will be positive and some negative, and the sum of the d's and that of the f's will both be zero. Then we multiply d_1 by f_1, preserving signs, and sum the n pairs of such products. This sum divided by $(n - 1)$ is the covariance. An example is given in table A.3. We shall denote the covariance between X and Y by "cov(X,Y)." If the true covariance is not zero, then X and Y are not independent. The converse, unfortunately, is not, in general, true, but at least the variates are then said to be uncorrelated.

• *Note that a correlation can exist only between two random variables.*

THE CORRELATION COEFFICIENT

It seems clear enough that whether or not X and Y are unrelated should not depend on the scales in which they are measured. If height in inches is unrelated to weight in pounds, reason demands that height in centimeters should be unrelated to weight in kilograms. Yet the covariance we have discussed is scale-dependent. One way of getting rid of this undesirable property is by rescaling everything in multiples of the standard deviation. The quantity

Table A.4. Short Method of Computing the Sample Covariance
and the Sample Correlation Coefficient from the Data in Table A.3

	x	y
Sample size	10	10
Sum of values	−26.48	−11.86
Sample means	−2.648	−1.186
Sample sum of squares	918.543,2	806.4626
[sum]^2/10 = [sum][mean]	70.119,040	14.065,960
Sum of squares from mean	848.424,160	792.396,640
Sample variance	94.269,351	88.044,071

Sum of the products of each x with its y = 91.140,300
Subtract the product of one total and the other mean, i.e.,
[−26.48][−1.186] = [−2.648][−11.86] = 31.405,280
To give the sum of the products of the deviations from the means = 59.735,020
Divide by the square root of the product of the residual sums of squares
= $\sqrt{[848.424,160][792.396,640]}$ = $\sqrt{672,288.4536}$ ... = 819.931 ...
    correlation coefficient = 59.735020/819.931 ... = 0.0729

$$r_{XY} = [\text{cov}(X,Y)]/\sqrt{[\text{var}(X)\text{var}(Y)]} \tag{4}$$

is known as the correlation coefficient. An example of the calculations is given in table A.4.

Properties of the Correlation Coefficient

1. The correlation coefficient has no meaning unless X and Y are *both random variables.* (For instance, it would be meaningless to compute it if X were, say, a dose of a drug that the investigator decided on rather than picking at random.)
2. The correlation coefficient is never less than −1 (perfect negative correlation) or more than +1 (perfect positive correlation).
3. A value of 0 means that the two variables are uncorrelated. If they follow the Gaussian distribution, then uncorrelatedness also means independence. *For distributions in general, however, these terms are not interchangeable.* It is quite possible for two variables to be perfectly dependent and to have a correlation coefficient of zero.
4. As we have noted, the correlation coefficient is unaffected by changes in scale or baseline.

THE GAUSSIAN ("NORMAL") DISTRIBUTION

Much of statistics centers on variables that follow this distribution. It has a technical description that would be out of place here.

Table A.5. Some Approximate Probabilities for the Gaussian Distribution

If the number of standard deviations that the sample value lies above the mean is	The area to the right of it and under the curve is approximately
1/3	2/5
2/3	1/4
1	1/6
4/3	1/11
5/3	1/21
2	1/44
7/3	1/100
8/3	1/260
3	1/740

For practical purposes, readers may be satisfied with the following rough checks for conformity to this distribution, especially if the sample is of large size and they are mainly concerned with statements about the mean of the distribution. The appropriate course is to divide the sample range up into ten to fifteen equal parts (depending on the size of the sample and the convenience of the intervals), find how many of the sample values fall in each interval, and draw a histogram. Then, at least roughly, we may expect a Gaussian variable to have the following properties:

1. There will be one clear mode.
2. The pattern will be more or less symmetrical about this mode.
3. The histogram will have tapered tails and a rounded central portion.
4. If the sample mean is located and the baseline marked off in multiples of the sample standard deviation, the proportions, besides being symmetrical about the mean, will follow the figures given in table A.5.

Some Properties of the Gaussian Variate

1. The sample mean and variance contain all the information that there is in the sample. (There is no need to be concerned about the mode, range, or any other statistic, and there is no point in recording sample estimates of them.)
2. For any example the reader is likely to meet, all weighted sums of Gaussian variates are Gaussian variates. This is true whether the quantities being summed have the same mean and vari-

ance, whether or not the weights are equal, and whether or not the variates are independent. It follows that the sample mean of a Gaussian variate is a Gaussian variate whatever the size of the sample. The mean for the sample mean will be the same as that for the parent distribution, and its variance will, of course, be σ^2/n, as in formula 2.

3. There is an interesting extension of the foregoing property. The sample means of a random sample of size n from *any* distribution (provided only that the variance is finite, as it will be for any natural set of measurements) will follow a Gaussian distribution approximately, and the larger n, the closer the fit. This remarkable property furnishes a justification for the widespread use of statistics based on Gaussian distributions even when the parent data are not Gaussian.

4. If two Gaussian variates are uncorrelated, they are also independent, and conversely.

5. The *standard normal distribution* is one rescaled in multiples of its standard deviation. Suppose that height in men is normally distributed with a mean of 175 cm and a standard deviation of 10 cm. A reading of 160 cm is 15 cm below the mean, which is 1.5 standard deviations below the mean. On the standard normal distribution, then, we represent its value by -1.5. In general, the standard normal form is given by subtracting the mean from the sample value and dividing by the standard deviation:

$$z = \frac{x - \mu}{\sigma} \tag{5}$$

This is the form given in table A.5.

THE CHI-SQUARE DISTRIBUTION

If Z, the standard normal variate, is squared, we might call it the Z-squared distribution. But for historical reasons it is called the "chi-square distribution with one degree of freedom," and is written χ_1^2. If any number—say n—of independent chi-square variates are added, the result is "a chi-square variate with n degrees of freedom." Its formula is somewhat complicated, but it is extensively tabled. The mean of a chi-square variate is its degrees of freedom, and its variance, twice its degrees of freedom. If n is large—say a hundred or more—the chi-square distribution is close to Gaussian; one may then convert the sample value (χ_n^2) into an approximate standard normal deviate by formula 5, as follows:

$$\frac{\chi_n^2 - n}{\sqrt{2n}},$$

and the result may be interpreted from table A.5.

THE BINOMIAL DISTRIBUTION

This distribution may be used wherever the outcomes from an experiment fulfill six conditions.

1. There are only two possible outcomes for each datum (e.g., living or dead; male or female; affected or unaffected).
2. Each datum is independent (we could, not, for instance, include twins as two separate data); and
3. At constant probabilities (We could not use it for mortality rates in an operation where some patients are weaker than others).
4. The results given to each datum are 1 ("success") or 0 ("failure"). (We could not, for instance, give a score of 2 to a patient who has survived a bilateral operation.) Note that the terms *failure* and *success* do not involve any statement of worthiness. For the attribute *sex*, it is of no importance whether we call maleness a success or a failure, provided that we do it in the same fashion throughout the study.
5. The results are added.
6. The number of subjects in the study is not a random variable but is fixed in advance. (There shall be no such thing as "quitting when you are ahead.")

If n subjects are studied under these conditions, and the (constant) probability of success for each is p, the binomial variate (i.e., the number of successes) has the mean value np and the variance of $np(1 - p)$. The mean proportion of successes is p, and the variance of the proportion is $p(1 - p)/n$. Tables exist for finding the individual terms in the binomial distribution; in general, however, if both np and $n(1 - p)$ exceed 10, one may use formula 5 to get the standard normal approximation:

$$z = \frac{x - np}{\sqrt{np(1 - p)}}.$$

Naturally, we might square this approximation and use the chi-square approximation instead

$$\chi_1^2 = \frac{(x - np)^2}{np(1 - p)}.$$

With a little maneuvering, we might rewrite this

$$\chi_1^2 = \frac{(x - np)^2}{np} + \frac{[(n - x) - n(1 - p)]^2}{n(1 - p)},\tag{6}$$

which may be conveniently remembered as computing for each class (in this case two, the failures and the successes) the quantity

$$\frac{(\text{Observed number} - \text{predicted number})^2}{\text{predicted number}}$$

and adding them. Note that although there are two classes, the number of degrees of freedom is still one.

Example A.1. Among twenty-five progeny of couples of whom one has familial polyposis coli, eight are affected, seventeen are not (124, pp. 288 ff). Test the Mendelian hypothesis that the probability of being affected is 1/2.

Under the null hypothesis, we predict $np = (25)(1/2) = n(1 - p)$ = 12.5 in each class. (The fact that half a person cannot be affected and that therefore the predicted value can never be attained does not matter.) The predicted variance is $np(1 - p) = 25(.5)(.5) = 6.25$, of which the square root (the standard deviation) is 2.5. Then the simple Gaussian approximation to the binomial test is

$$z = (8 - 12.5)/2.5 = -1.8,$$

which being greater than 1.645, would lead to rejection of the hypothesis at the 10 percent level. If we square this, to get 3.24, and match it against the chi-square distribution with one degree of freedom, we arrive at exactly the same conclusion. If we use alternative formula 6, we get

$$\chi_1^2 = \frac{(8 - 12.5)^2}{12.5} + \frac{(17 - 12.5)^2}{12.5},$$

which gives exactly the same result.

THE MULTINOMIAL DISTRIBUTION

This is a generalization of the binomial. Instead of two outcomes (success and failure), there may be three or more, e.g., healthy, sick, and dead, or single, married, widowed, and divorced. The operations carry over without a hitch. Obviously, the sum of the probabilities of these individual and mutually exclusive outcomes must add to unity, or the categorization is not exhaustive. (For each unit in the sample, some outcome is certain to happen.) The predicted number in each will be the product of the probability and the sample size. The chi-square test is done by using formula 6. However, the number of terms to be summed will depend on the number of classes. The number of degrees of freedom is found as follows:

1. Count one degree of freedom for each category.
2. Subtract one degree of freedom for each distinct constraint.
3. Subtract one degree of freedom for each distinct unknown parameter that has to be estimated *from the present sample* in order to determine the predicted values.

NOTES

1. By a constraint, we mean a limitation imposed on how the data must behave. For instance, there may be four classes in a sample: affected and unaffected members of the two sexes. By fixing the sample size at 100, we have imposed a constraint and there are three degrees of freedom left after we have taken one (for the constraint) from the number of classes (four). But if we require the numbers of men and women in the sample to be 50 each, we have imposed two constraints and there are only two degrees of freedom left.

2. If (as in example A.1) the proportion we expect to be affected is a constitutive parameter (that is, one that arises from the genetic nature of the problem), we do not need to estimate it. But if we had the hypothesis to test that the proportion of affected is the same in males as in females, and for lack of other leads we had to estimate the proportion affected by taking, say, 8/25, then the test would have one degree of freedom less as a result, i.e., in the present case, 2. If, further, we were not prepared to suppose that the probability of a progeny picked at random being male is 1/2 and we estimated this parameter as well, then we would have only one degree of freedom left. (This latter type of case where the proportions are estimated from the data is called a *contingency table*.)

3. Certain stereotyped cases have well-known answers. The commonest is the two-way multiple classification traditionally represented by r rows, and c columns. (For instance, one might group the data in four ways by marital status and three ways by political opinion. This is a 4×3 contingency table.) Assuming that all the proportions have to be estimated from the data, the number of degrees of freedom is $(r - 1)(c - 1)$, in this case $(3)(2) = 6$.

Glossary

Accurate: (used of an estimator) unbiased or nearly unbiased.

Alleles: genes that differ in detail but compete with each other to occupy the same genetic locus.

Aptness: (used of a hypothesis or surmise) conformity to the empirical facts.

Asymmetry: see *Skewness*.

Asymptotic: used of a relationship between a variable and a quantity or property that is more nearly attained as the variable becomes more extreme.

Authentication (principle of): a statement may be said to be false only if it could conceivably be shown to be true if it is true. (Cf. *Falsifiability, principle of; Verification.*)

Bias: any trend in the collection, analysis, interpretation, publication, or review of data that leads to conclusions systematically different from the truth.

Binomial: having two possible outcomes. ——— **distribution:** a discrete distribution representing the number of outcomes out of a fixed number of identical, independent, ——— events that are of a particular type. (See Appendix for details.)

Canon: an established rule, to be changed only formally and with reluctance, that prescribes how a process (e.g., a proof) shall be properly carried out. (It is akin to Kuhn's term *paradigm*, which is, however, conceptual rather than methodological.)

Circadian: having a regular cycle, one cycle being completed every twenty-four hours.

Confidence limits: a set of values, furnished by an analysis that may be said with a specified degree of assurance to encompass the true value of an unknown parameter.

Confounding: a relationship between the effects of two or more causal factors as observed in a set of data, such that it is not logically possible to infer the contribution of any cause to an effect.

Consistent: (used of an estimator) giving an answer that is more and more certain to be close to the true value as the sample size increases.

Criterion: a bench mark invoked to gauge the soundness of a conclusion.

Decision theory: a branch of statistics concerned with discerning and using the factors that bear on the making of decisions that will have preassigned properties.

Deduction: a type of argument that proceeds from the general to the particular. Soundly used, it is logically compelling, but it has only limited scope in science. (Contrast with *Induction.*)

Deterministic: brought to completion without the intervention of chance.

Efficient: (used of a consistent estimator) having a small variance. **Absolutely ———:** having the smallest variance possible among consistent estimators.

Empirical: concerned with finding answers by appeal to observation and experiment rather than to reasoning alone.

Epistasis: genetic interaction between nonalleles—especially the hiding of the phenotype of the one by the other.

Estimate: a formal guess made from random data about the value of a parameter.

Estimation: a branch of statistics concerned with devising estimators (q.v.) that provides a method of freely choosing values of a parameter that have certain desirable properties. (Contrast with *Hypothesis testing.*)

Estimator: a recipe for systematically extracting an estimate from data.

Etiology: the empirical study of the causative ingredients of a disease. (Contrast with *Pathogenesis.*)

Falsifiability (principle of): a statement may be said to be true only if it could be shown to be false, if false. (Cf. *Authentication, principle of; Verification.*)

Galtonian: a system, especially genetic, in which the outcome is determined by many separate components that all have more or less equal, independent, and additive effects. (Its quantitative effect is well approximated by the Gaussian distribution.)

Gaussian: used of a particular, continuous distribution that is symmetrical and unimodal and has no finite limits. It is an approximation for many distributions, such as the binomial, and for many processes, such as the Galtonian.

Heterozygous: used of a state of an organism in which the two alleles at a Mendelian locus differ from one another.

Histogram: a visual display of data, empirical or theoretical, on a random variable in which, by convention, each reading is represented as a rectangle of unvarying size located on an ascending scale of the value of the random variable. (See figs. 4.1 and 4.5 as examples.)

Homozygous: used of a state of an organism in which the two alleles at a Mendelian locus are identical.

Hypothesis: any conjecture cast in a form that will allow it to be verified.

Hypothesis testing: a statistical procedure for deciding whether or not a set of random data can be plausibly accounted for by a distribution with conjectured parameters. (Contrast with *Estimation*.)

Illation: a form of advance in understanding of a scientific process in which the investigator cannot appeal to formal deduction or inference or to assured prior principles of either. Taking a (usually small) "leap in the dark."

Incidence: the rate at which an event occurs per unit time per person in the members of a defined population at risk.

Induction: a type of argument from particular and unstructured experiences to general conclusions about a population. **Mathematical ———:** argument step by step from the relationship between consecutive pairs of an ordered set, and hence to all members of the set.

Inference: that branch of formal scientific argumentation that is concerned with reaching conclusions about the parameters of a specified process from empirical evidence and on the basis of axioms and criteria that are reached independently of the data and are not open to question during the course of the process. (Contrast with *Illation; Probability algebra*.)

Locus (genetic): the part or homologous parts of a genome that may be occupied by any of a set of *alleles*.

Mean: (also called the expectation) the average value of a *variate* (q.v.).

Median: the fiftieth *percentile* of a distribution.

Mendelian: dealing with the genetics of the individual genetic locus in isolation. (Contrast with *Galtonian*.)

Metastasis: (of a cancer) spread to a distant site as fragments borne in blood or other fluid, as distinct from direct spread by growth. The tissue so spread (also called a secondary).

Modality: the number of modes exhibited by a *histogram* or *probability distribution*. (Multiple modes are somewhat precariously taken as evidence of heterogeneity.)

Mode: (of a distribution) that value of the *variate* at which there is a higher concentration of probability (or, empirically, of cases) than at any point in its immediate neighborhood.

Model: an abstract representation of the relationship between logical, analytical, or empirical components of a system. Usually it involves some sacrifice of authentic detail to tractability and coherence.

Monotonic: a variable, Y, is a monotonic function of a variable, X, if an increase in X, however small, is always associated with a change in Y that is of constant sign. If the change in Y also is always positive, Y is a monotonic increasing function; if it is negative, it is monotonic decreasing.

Null hypothesis: a *hypothesis* set up for empirical testing that, if not thereby shown untenable, will (provisionally, at least) be accepted as true.

Objective: the goal that is being pursued in a field of organized enquiry. (Not to be confused with a *canon* or a *criterion*. The objective of therapeutic oncology is to cure cancer. The canon is empirical experience. The criterion is demonstrated increase in survival, relief of pain, etc.)

Outcome variable: See *Regression*.

Paradigm: a pattern of thought or conceptualization. (Cf. *Canon*.)

Paralytic ileus: a state (commonly postoperative or due to peritonitis) in which the intestine lies inert, without the contractions that occur from time to time in a normal bowel.

Parameter: a quantity of statistical interest that may vary, but not randomly. (Contrast with *Variate*.)

Pathogenesis: the process whereby the etiological causative ingredients produce a disease.

Pentheric: a property (of a solution to a problem) that, though obtrusive, is incidental to the main purpose. (A surgeon is required to wear a sterile operating gown. The *color* of the gown has nothing to do with its sterility, although a pentheric tradition requires it to be white or green.)

Percentile: the kth percentile of a distribution is that value of the variate such that there is a probability of $k/100$ that it will equal or exceed a randomly chosen value of the variate.

Plausibility: that aspect of a hypothesis or surmise that appeals to native common sense and general knowledge rather than to formal analysis. (Contrast with *Aptness*.)

Poisson distribution: the distribution of the number of discrete events that occur in unit time provided that the probability of an event occurring within any interval of fixed length is constant, and independent of the occurrence of any other event.

Population: (also universe or reference set): a group of elements sharing common qualities, about which it is in some sense considered worthwhile to predicate corporate properties.

Power: used of a test of a statistical hypothesis to denote the probability that a hypothesis will be rejected if it is indeed false.

Precise: used of an estimator that has a low standard deviation but is not necessarily *accurate* (q.v.).

Prevalence: the frequency of a trait in a population. **Point ———:** the proportion of a population that exhibits the trait at a particular instant. **Term ———:** the proportion of the population that exhibits the trait for at least part of a specified interval of time.

Probability algebra: that branch of formal argumentation that deals with predictions of the outcome of a stochastic process from an agreed set of axioms. (Contrast with *Illation; Inference*.)

Probability distribution: a predictive statement about a single future outcome of a random process, comprising three entities: a random variable; the set of all possible values that it may assume; and the probability (or probability density) associated with each.

Proband: that member of a cluster through whom the cluster is brought to the attention of an investigator. (For example, in genetics, the cluster would be a family; in infectious disease, it is often a household.)

Random sampling: a method of selecting a subset of a population such that the probability of any particular subset being selected may be specified in advance.

Reference set: see *Population*.

Regression: a graded relationship by which the distribution of the outcome of a random process (the **outcome variable**) may be more precisely described from information given by another quantity (the **regressor variable**), and from which it is to be predicted.

Robust: used of a statistical procedure that is not exquisitely sensitive to departures from the assumptions on which it is strictly predicated.

Significance level: an evaluation, *after the fact*, of the size of a test of hypothesis (see following entry) such that, if it had been chosen in advance, would barely have led to the rejection of the null statistical hypothesis.

Size of a test of hypothesis: the risk, *chosen in advance,* that the analyst is prepared to take that the null hypothesis will be declared false when it is, in fact, true. (The size of the test is not to be confused with the size of the sample used in the test.)

Skepsis: the cultivation of an incisive attitude toward the cogency of data put forward against, or in support of, a theory.

Skepticism: the attitude that, in the nature of things, it is impossible, even undesirable, to attain certainty about any proposition.

Skewness: (used of a distribution) asymmetry. A variate is commonly said to be positively skewed if the *mean* and the *median* exceed the *mode* (qq.v.).

Standard deviation: the (positive) square root of the variance.

Statistics: the formal principles of interpreting empirical scientific data, in the light of *given canons of enquiry,* and comprising mainly *hypothesis testing* and *inference* (qq.v). (Contrast with *Illation; Probability algebra.*)

Stochastic: probabilistic (usually used of an event taking place in time or distance). (Contrast with *Deterministic.*)

Strategic: used of the large-scale, rather coarse-grained plans of an enquiry or policy ("the big picture"). (Contrast with *Tactical.*)

Sufficiency: 1. Used of a cause or condition that guarantees a particular conclusion. ("Depriving a child of oxygen for an hour is a sufficient cause of death"). 2. Used of a statistic that contains all the information (about a particular parameter) that is contained in a sample.

Systemic: a term applied to a mode of action (of a drug, treatment, etc.) that is determined, not by anatomical location, but by similarity of function or metabolism.

Tactical: used of detailed, rather than broad, plans. (Contrast with *Strategic.*)

Tautology: a statement or proposition that by its nature can, and need, be neither authenticated nor falsified. (All identities and definitions are tautologous.)

Translocation: (in genetics) the breaking off of a fragment of chromosome and the reattachment of it elsewhere in the genome. The resulting chromosomes of such processes. **Balanced ———:** an assembly of chromosomes exhibiting one or more ——— such that the normal genetic content is contained (but rearranged) in each cell.

Transposition of the viscera: a congenital anomaly in which asymmetrical structures of the body are located on the side opposite that which they usually occupy (e.g., the liver and appendix on the left; the spleen and heart on the right).

Universe: see *Population.*

Validation: the process of establishing that a method of argumentation is sound. (Contrast with *Verification,* which deals with truth of conclusions and with which it is often confused.)

Variable: used of a formal quantity that may take on any of a set of values (known as the domain of the variable).

Variance: the mean value of the square of the distance of a variable from the mean of the distribution.

Variate: (or random variable): a variable that may assume any of a set of values, each with a preassigned probability (known as its distribution).

Verification: the process of testing whether a set of data, a surmise, or a proposition is true. (Not to be confused with *validation,* which is a process applied to methods. A method may be sound, but a conclusion false, and conversely. That is, an argument may be valid but the conclusions false—for instance, because the axioms are false.) **Principle of ————:** the criterion that to assert that a statement is true, there must be some method external to the statement that corroborates it. (Cf. *Tautology.*)

References

1. Murphy, E. A. "The analysis and interpretation of experiments: Philosophical issues." *J Med and Philo* 7:307–25, 1982.
2. Schlosstein, L., Terasaki, P. I., Bluestone, R., and Pearson, C. M. "High association of an HL-A antigen, W27, with ankylosing spondylitis." *New Eng J Med* 288:704–6, 1973.
3. Smythe, H., Ogryzlo, M. A., Murphy, E. A., and Mustard, J. F. "The effects of sulphinpyrazone (Anturan) on platelet economy and blood coagulation in man." *Canad Med Ass J* 92:818–21, 1965.
4. Mustard, J. F., Rowsell, H. C., Smythe, H. A., Senyi, A., and Murphy, E. A. "The effects of sulphinpyrazone on platelet economy and thrombus formation in rabbits." *Blood* 24:859–66, 1967.
5. Russell, B. *An Enquiry into Meaning and Truth*. London: Unwin, 1950.
6. Rosenhan, D. L. "On being sane in insane places." *Science* 179:250–58, 1973.
7. Rosenhan, D. L. "The contextual nature of psychiatric diagnosis." *Amer J Abnorm Psych* 84:462–74, 1975.
8. Pearson, K. "On the criterion that a given system of deviations from the probable in the case of a correlated system of variables is such that it can reasonably be supposed to have arisen from random sampling." *Phil Mag* 1:157–75, 1900. Reprinted in *Karl Pearson's Early Statistical Papers*. London: Cambridge University Press, 1948.
9. Yule, G. U., and Greenwood, M. "The statistics of antityphoid and anticholeric inoculation and the interpretation of such statistics in general." *Proc Roy Soc Med* 8:113 (epidemiological section), 1915.
10. Fisher, R. A. "On the interpretation of χ^2 from contingency tables and the calculation of P." *J Roy Stat Soc* 85 (pt. 1):87–94, 1922.
11. Murphy, E. A. *The Logic of Medicine*. Baltimore: Johns Hopkins University Press, 1976.
12. Murphy, E. A. *Skepsis, Dogma, and Belief: Uses and Abuses in Medicine*. Baltimore: Johns Hopkins University Press, 1981, Appendix.

13. Murphy, E. A. "Quantitative genetics: A critique." *Soc Biol* 23:126–41, 1980.
14. McKusick, V. A. *Mendelian Inheritance in Man.* Baltimore: Johns Hopkins University Press, sixth edition, 1983.
15. Velican, D., and Velican, C. "Studies of fibrous plaques occurring in the coronary arteries of children." *Atherosclerosis* 33:201–15, 1979.
16. Veatch, R. M. *A Theory of Medical Ethics.* New York: Basic Books, 1981, pp. 190–91.
17. Murphy, E. A., and Trojak, J. E. "The mutational debt: How is it paid?" in *Population and Biological Aspects of Human Mutation* (I. A. Porter and E. S. Hook, editors). New York: Academic Press, 1981, pp. 23–33.
18. Murphy, E. A., and Krush, A. J. "Familial polyposis coli" in *Progress in Medical Genetics* (A. G. Steinberg, A. G. Bearn, and B. Childs, editors). Philadelphia: Saunders, 1980, vol. 4, pp. 59–101.
19. Thompson, E. A., and Cannings, C. "Sampling schemes and ascertainment" in *Genetic Analysis of Common Disease: Applications to Predictive Factors in Coronary Disease* (C. F. Sing and M. Skolnick, editors). New York: Alan Liss, 1979, pp. 363–82.
20. Thorn, G. W. Personal communication.
21. Murphy, E. A. "Genetic and evolutionary fitness." *Am J Med Genet* 2:51–79, 1978.
22. Li, C. C. *Human Genetics: Principles and Methods.* New York: McGraw-Hill, 1961, pp. 145–46.
23. Lewis, C. S. *That Hideous Strength.* New York: Macmillan, 1946.
24. Lyon, M. F. "X-chromosome inactivation and developmental patterns in mammals." *Biological Reviews of the Cambridge Philosophical Society,* 47:1–25, 1972.
25. Macfarlane, R. G. "An enzyme cascade in the blood clotting mechanism and its function as a biochemical amplifier." *Nature* 202:498–99, 1964.
26. Whitehead, A. N. *Science and the Modern World.* New York: Macmillan, 1925.
27. Murphy, E. A., Krush, A. J., Dietz, M., and Rhode, C. A. "Hereditary polyposis coli III: Genetic and evolutionary fitness." *Amer J Hum Genet* 32:700–713, 1980.
28. Montegriffo, V. M. E. "Height and weight of a United Kingdom adult population with a review of anthropometric literature." *Ann Hum Genet (Lond.)* 31:389–99, 1968.
29. Smith, C. A. B. "Some comments on the statistical methods in linkage investigations." *Amer J Hum Genet* 11:289–304, 1959.
30. Melnick, E. L., and Tenenbein, A. "Misspecifications of the normal distribution." *Amer Statistician* 36:372–73, 1982.
31. Fried, K., and Davies, A. M. "Some effects on the offspring of uncle-niece marriages in the Moroccan Jewish Community in Jerusalem." *Amer J Hum Genet* 26:65–72, 1974.

32. Haldane, J. B. S. "A method of investigating recessive characters in man." *J Genet* 25:251–57, 1932.
33. Fisher, R. A. "Has Mendel's work been rediscovered?" *Annals Science* 1:115–37, 1936.
34. Lilienfeld, A. M. "A methodological problem in testing a recessive genetic hypothesis in human disease." *Amer J Public Health* 49:199–204, 1959.
35. Murphy, E. A., and Chase, G. A. *Principles of Genetic Counseling.* Chicago: Year Book, 1975.
36. Emery, A. E. H. *Methodology in Medical Genetics: An Introduction to Statistical Methods.* Churchill Livingstone: Edinburgh, 1976.
37. Kelly, T. E. *Clinical Genetics and Genetic Counseling.* Chicago: Year Book, 1980.
38. LaDue, J. S., Murison, P. J., and Pack, G. T. "The use of tetraethylammonium bromide as a diagnostic test in pheochromocytoma." *Ann Int Med* 29:914–21, 1948.
39. Robertson, D., Goldberg, M., Hollister, A. S., Wade, D., and Robertson, M. R. "Clonidine raises blood pressure in severe idiopathic orthostatic hypotension." *Amer J Med* 74:193–200, 1983.
40. Zaimis, E. "The interruption of ganglionic transmission and some of its problems." *J Pharm Pharmacol* 7:497–511, 1955. Mannegazza, P., Tyler, C., and Zaimis, E. "The peripheral action of hexamethonium and pentolinium." *Brit J Pharmacol* 13:480–84, 1958.
41. Renie, W. A., and Murphy, E. A. "The dynamics of quantifiable homeostasis: II. Characterization of linear processes." *Amer J Med Genet* 15:637–53, 1983.
42. Murphy, E. A., and Trojak, J. E. "The genetics of quantifiable homeostasis: 1. The individual." *Amer J Med Genet* 15:275–90, 1983.
43. Leder, P. "The genetics of antibody diversity." *Sci Amer* 246:5, 102–15, 1982.
44. Fabre, J. H. *Bramble-Bees and Others* (translated by A. T. de Mattos). New York: Dodd Mead, 1915.
45. von Frisch, K. *Bees: Their Vision, Chemical Senses, and Language.* Cornell: Cornell University Press, 1950.
46. Murphy, E. A. "Detection of genetic effects of environmental agents." *Envir Health Perspect* 42:127–36, 1981.
47. Murphy, E. A. "The genetic dynamics of disease." *Am J Med Genet* 8:35–52, 1981.
48. McKusick, V. A., Egeland, J. A., Eldridge, R., and Krusen, D. E. "Dwarfism in the Amish: 1. The Ellis van Creveld syndrome." *Bull Johns Hopkins Hosp* 115:306–36, 1964.
49. von Willebrand, E. A. "Über hereditäre Pseudohemophilie." *Acta Med Scand* 76:521–50, 1931.
50. Finucci, J. M., and Childs, B. "Dyslexia: Family Studies" in *Genetic Aspects of Speech and Language Disorders* (C. L. Ludlow and J. A. Cooper, editors). New York: Academic Press, 1983, pp. 157–67.

51. Silverman, W. H. "The lesson of retrolental fibroplasia." *Scient Amer* 236:100–107, June 1977.
52. Wintrobe, M. M., and others. *Clinical Hematology*. Philadelphia: Lea and Febiger, seventh edition, 1974, pp. 602–10.
53. Fraser, D. W., and McDade, J. E. "Legionellosis." *Scient Amer* 241:81–99, Oct 1977.
54. Ingram, V. M. "Abnormal human haemoglobin: III. The chemical difference between normal and sickle-cell haemoglobin." *Biochim Biophys Acta* 36:402–11, 1959.
55. Williams, R. R. *Towards the Conquest of Beriberi*. Cambridge, Mass.: Harvard University Press, 1961.
56. Koch, R. "The aetiology of tuberculosis" (translated by B. Pinner and M. Pinner). *Amer Rev Tuberc* 25:298–323, 1932.
57. Goldstein, J. L., and Brown, M. S. "The LDL receptor defect in familial hypercholesterolemia." *Med Clin N Amer* 66, no. 2:335–62, 1982.
58. Cannon, W. B. *The Wisdom of the Body*. New York: Norton, 1932.
59. Bernard, C. *De la physiologie générale*. Paris: Hachette, 1872.
60. Lerner, I. M. *Genetic Homeostasis*. Edinburgh: Oliver and Body, 1954.
61. Waddington, C. H. *The Strategy of the Genes*. London: Allen and Unwin, 1957.
62. Moore, S, ed. *Vascular Injury and Atherosclerosis*. New York: Marcel Dekker, 1981.
63. Armitage, P., and Doll, R. "A two-stage theory of carcinogenesis in relation to the age distribution of human cancer." *Brit J Cancer* 9:161–69, 1957.
64. Moolgavkar, S. H., Day, N. E., and Stevens, R. G. "Two-stage model for carcinogenesis: Epidemiology of breast cancer in females." *J Nat Cancer Inst* 65:559–69, 1980. Moolgavkar, S. H., and Knudson, A. G. "Mutation and cancer: A model for human carcinogenesis." *JNCI* 66:1037–52, 1981.
65. Knudson, A. G. "Mutation and childhood cancer: A probability model for the incidence of retinoblastoma." *Proc Nat Acad Sci* 72:5116–20, 1975.
66. Wilson, E. B. "The sex chromosomes." *Archiv Microsk Anat* 77:249–71, 1911.
67. McKusick, V. A. *Heritable Disorders of Connective Tissue*. Mosby: St. Louis, fourth edition, 1972.
68. Kety, S. S., and Schmidt, C. F. "The determination of cerebral blood flow in man by the use of nitrous oxide in low concentrations." *Amer J Physiol* 143:53–56, 1945.
69. Gale, A. N., and Murphy, E. A. "The use of serum creatine phosphokinase in genetic counseling for Duchenne muscular dystrophy: I. Analysis of results from twenty-nine studies." *J Chron Dis* 31: 101–9, 1978. "II. Review of methods of assay and factors which may be

relevant in the interpretation of serum creatine phosphokinase activity." ibid. 32:639–51, 1979.

70. Kuhn, T. S. *The Structure of Scientific Revolutions*. Chicago: University of Chicago Press, second edition, 1970.

71. Pauling, L., and Corey, R. B. "Atomic coordinates and structure factors for the helical configurations of polypeptide chains." *PNAS* 37:235–40, 1951. "The structure of synthetic polypeptides." ibid., pp. 241–50. "The pleated sheet, a new layer configuration of polypeptide chains." ibid., pp. 251–56. "The structure of feather rachis keratin." ibid., pp. 256–61. "The structure of hair, muscle, and related proteins." ibid., pp. 261–71. "The structure of fibrous proteins of the collagen-gelatin group." ibid., pp. 272–81. "The polypeptide-chain configuration in hemoglobin and other globular proteins." ibid., pp. 282–85.

72. Murphy, E. A., Rosell, E. M., and Rosell, M. I. "Deduction, inference, and illation." Unpublished analysis.

73. Wiener, N. *Cybernetics, or Control and Communication in the Animal and the Machine*. New York: Wiley, 1948.

74. Dunn, L. C. *A Short History of Genetics: The Development of Some of the Main Lines of Thought, 1864–1939*. New York: McGraw-Hill, 1965.

75. Fisher, R. A. *The Genetic Theory of Natural Selection*. Oxford: Oxford University Press, 1930. Revised version New York: Dover, 1958.

76. Chargaff, E. "Chemical specificity of nucleic acids and mechanism of their enzymatic degradation." *Experientia* 6:201–9, 1950.

77. Watson, J. H., and Crick, F. H. C. "Genetic implications of the structure of deoxyribosenucleic acid." *Nature* 171:964–67, 1953.

78. Lejeune, J., Gautier, M., and Turpin, M. R. "Etude des chromosomes somatiques de neuf enfants mongoliens." *C R Acad Sci Paris* 248:1721–22, 1959.

79. Ellis, C. *Bost Med Surg J* 90:13–14, 1874. (Untitled case report.)

80. Damoiseau, L-H-C. *Du diagnostic et du traitement de la pleurésie*. Paris, n.p., 1845.

81. Kaunitz, J. "Liquid levels and other liquid surfaces in pleural effusions." *J Thoracic Surgery* 4:300–309, 1935.

82. Davis, S., Gardner, E., and Qvist, G. "The shape of a pleural effusion." *Brit Med J* i pp. 436–37, 1963.

83. Polya, G. *Mathematics and Plausible Reasoning*. Princeton: Princeton University Press, 1954.

84. Welch, W. H., in *System of Medicine* (T. C. Allbutt, editor). London: Macmillan, 1892, vol. 6, pp. 155 ff.

85. Hamilton, M., Thompson, E. N., and Wisniewski, T. K. M. "The role of blood-pressure control in preventing complications of hypertension." *Lancet* i, pp. 235–38, 1964.

86. Freis, E. D., and associates. "Effects of treatment on morbidity in hypertension." *J Amer Med Ass* 202:1028–34, 1967.

87. Longford, E. *Victoria R. I.* London: Weidenfeld and Nicolson, 1971, p. 69.

88. Rufer, V., Bauer, J., and Soukup, F. "On the heredity of eye color." *Acta Univ Carol Med* 16:429–34, 1970.

89. Reed, T. E. "Red hair colour as a genetical character." *Ann Eugen* 17:115–39, 1952.

90. Baker, G. A. "Transformations of bimodal distributions." *Ann Math Stat* 1:334–44, 1930.

91. Murphy, E. A. "Classification and its alternatives" in *Clinical Judgment: A Critical Appraisal* (Engelhard , H. T., Spicker, S. F., and Towers, B., editors). Dordrecht, Holland: Reidel, 1979, pp. 59–85.

92. Lewis, T. *Diseases of the Heart and Circulation: Described for Practitioners and Students.* New York: MacMillan, 1934.

93. Popper, K. R. *Conjectures and Refutations: The Growth of Scientific Knowledge.* New York: Harper and Row, 1963.

94. Popper, K. R. *The Logic of Scientific Discovery.* New York: Harper and Row, 1959.

95. Selyi, H. "A syndrome produced by diverse nocuous agents." *Nature* 138:32, 1936. "The general adaptation syndrome and the diseases of adaptation." *J Clin Endocrin Metab.* 6:117–30. 1946.

96. Murphy, E. A. *Probability in Medicine.* Baltimore: Johns Hopkins University Press, 1979.

97. Wintrobe, M. M., and others: *Clinical Hematology.* Philadelphia: Lea and Febiger, seventh edition, 1974, pp. 115–19.

98. Fischer, S. L., and Fischer, S. P. "Mean corpuscular volume." *Arch Int Med* 143:282–83, 1983.

99. Kimball, A. W. "Errors of the third kind in statistical consulting." *J Amer Stat Ass* 52:133–42, 1957.

100. Macklin, M. T. "Inheritance of retinoblastoma in Ohio." *Arch Ophthalmol* 62:842–51, 1959.

101. Ramon y Cajal, S. *Histologie du Système Nerveux.* Madrid: Consejo Superior de Investigaciones Cientificas, 1952.

102. Barr, M. L., Bertram, L. F., and Lindsay, H. A. "The morphology of the nerve cell nucleus according to sex." *Anat Rev* 107:283–97, 1950.

103. Waardenburg, P. J. *Das Menschliche Auge und seine Erbanlagen.* The Hague: Martinus Nijhoff, 1932.

104. Bleyer, A. "Indications that mongolian imbecility is a gametic mutation of degenerative type." *Am J Dis Child* 47:342–48, 1934.

105. Nordling, C. O. "A new theory on the cancer-inducing mechanism." *Brit J Cancer* 7:68–72, 1953.

106. Fisher, J. C., and Hollomon, J. H. "A hypothesis for the origin of cancer foci." *Cancer* 4:916–18, 1951.

107. Muller, H. J. "Artificial transmutation of the gene." *Science* 66:84–87, 1927.

108. Matsunaga, E. "Hereditary retinoblastoma: Delayed mutation or host resistance?" *Amer J Hum Genet* 30:406–24, 1978.

109. Murphy, E. A. "The pursuit of the minor premise: A commentary on normality." *Metamedicine* 2:283–99, 1981.

110. Vogel, F., and Motulsky, A. G. *Human Genetics: Problems and Approaches.* New York: Springer, 1979, p. 246.

111. Galton, F. *Natural Inheritance.* London: MacMillan, 1889.

112. Fisher, R. A. "The correlation between relatives on the supposition of Mendelian inheritance." *Trans Roy Soc Edin* 52:399–433, 1918.

113. Dahl, L. K., Heine, M., and Tassinari, L. "Effects of chronic excess salt ingestion." *J Exp Med* 115:1173–90, 1962.

114. Rapp, J. P., and Dahl, L. K. "Mutant forms of cytochrome P-450 controlling both 8- and 11-hydroxylation in the rat." *Biochemistry* 15:1235–42, 1976.

115. Fraser, F. C. "Evolution of a palatable multifactorial threshold model." *Amer J Hum Genet* 32:796–813, 1978.

116. Murphy, E. A., Trojak, J. E., Hou, W., and Rohde, C. A. "The bingo model of survivorship: 1. Probabilistic aspects." *Amer J Med Genet* 10:261–77, 1981.

117. Levine, P., Robinson, E., Celano, M., Briggs, O., and Falkinburg, L. "Gene interaction resulting in suppression of blood group substance B." *Blood* 10:1100–1108, 1955.

118. Penrose, L. S. *An Introduction to Human Biochemical Genetics.* Eugen Lab Memoirs XXXVII. London: Cambridge University Press, 1955.

119. Arieti, S. "Schizophrenia: The manifest symptomatology, the psychodynamic and formal mechanisms," chapter 23 in *American Handbook of Psychiatry, vol. 1* (S. Arieti, editor). New York: Basic Books, 1959. See especially the section on Paleologic thought (pp. 478–79).

120. Elsom, K. O., Ipsem, J., Clark, T. W., Talerica, L., and Yamagawa, H. "Physicians' use of objective data in clinical diagnosis." *J Amer Med Ass* 201:109–16, 1967.

121. Eddington, A. S. *The Nature of the Physical World.* London: Cambridge University Press, 1928.

122. Dixon, W. J., and Massey F. J. *Introduction to Statistical Analysis.* New York: McGraw-Hill, third edition, 1969.

123. Colton, T. *Statistics in Medicine.* Boston: Little Brown, 1975.

124. Murphy, E. A. *Biostatistics in Medicine.* Baltimore: Johns Hopkins University Press, 1982.

Index

About the Author

Edmond A. Murphy, M.D., is professor of medicine and head
of the Division of Medical Genetics at the Johns Hopkins
University. He is author of *Skepsis, Dogma, and Belief* and a
triology on the principles of interpreting empirical evidence
in clinical science: *The Logic of Medicine; Probability in Medicine;*
and *Biostatistics in Medicine.*

THE JOHNS HOPKINS UNIVERSITY PRESS

A Companion to Medical Statistics

This book was set in Baskerville text and Spartan display type
by the Composing Room of Michigan, Inc., from a design
by Cynthia W. Hotvedt.

It was printed on 50-lb Glatfelter Offset paper and bound in
Kivar by Thomson-Shore, Inc., Dexter, Michigan.

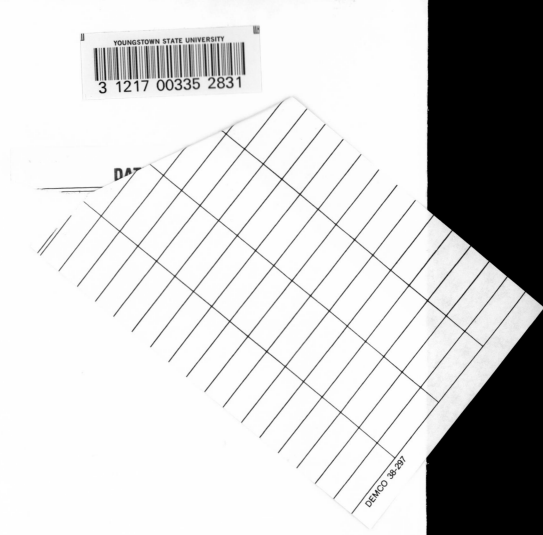

MAR 24 1987